MW01291540

ARE YOU REALLY
LISTENING?

BERNICE SIMPSON

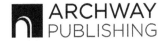
ARCHWAY
PUBLISHING

Archway Publishing books may be ordered through booksellers or by contacting:

Archway Publishing
1663 Liberty Drive
Bloomington, IN 47403
www.archwaypublishing.com
844-669-3957

NIV:
• Scripture quotations taken from The Holy Bible, New International Version® NIV® Copyright © 1973 1978 1984 2011 by Biblica, Inc. TM. Used by permission. All rights reserved worldwide.
NKJV:
• Scripture taken from the New King James Version® Copyright © 1982 by Thomas Nelson. Used by permission. All rights reserved.
KJV:
• Scripture taken from the King James Version of the Bible.
NLT:
• Scripture quotations marked (NLT) are taken from the Holy Bible, New Living Translation, copyright ©1996, 2004, 2015 by Tyndale House Foundation. Used by permission of Tyndale House Publishers, a Division of Tyndale House Ministries, Carol Stream, Illinois 60188. All rights reserved.

Interior Image Credit: Alexandra Hartwell, Keri Kubota, Tiara Butler

New International Version,King James Version, NLT 28

ISBN: 978-1-6657-3271-0 (sc)
ISBN: 978-1-6657-3270-3 (hc)
ISBN: 978-1-6657-3269-7 (e)

Library of Congress Control Number: 2022920076

Print information available on the last page.

Archway Publishing rev. date: 11/14/2022

PREFACE

This book is intended for nursing students or anyone who is curious about end-of-life experiences. Keep in mind that each person has his or her own way of exiting this world. I wanted to share some of the events that occurred during my twenty-nine-year career as a nurse.

Most patients' names have been changed to protect them—with the exception of Mrs. Beverly Goveart and her daughters, Vikki and Debbie, as well as Barbara Michael, Garnett Hawkins, Laura Truitt, George Wright, Larry Wright, Tanita Wright, Felecia Spalding, Renee Linton, Father Hayden, and Reverend Daly, who gave me consent to use their real names. The events described in this book are real.

Catherine Proppe gave consent to use citations from her book, *Greek Alphabet: Unlock the Secrets.*

Effective communication is essential in any conversation, but when a person is hospitalized, it is even more vital. Body language is a form of nonverbal communication that speaks volumes about your mindset when you enter a room.

"A letter from the heart can be read on the face."
~Swahili proverb

We can all be distracted at times, but active listening is key. Just remember to have patience and remain focused on your plan of care. Also, things do not always happen as systematically described in our nursing books. But then again, that is what makes nursing so interesting and challenging. End of life is significant because it is our last time to assist our patients or family members with completing a task before they depart from this Earth.

I have also incorporated stories about Ayurvedic treatments. Ayurveda is one of the world's oldest holistic (whole body) healing systems that emphasizes good health, prevention, and treatment of illness. *Ayurveda* translates to "knowledge of life," which encourages balance between body, mind, spirit, and environment.

When traditional medicine is used, it is extremely important to notify your primary care physician of any use of medications or herbal remedies, which includes over-the-counter medications related to potential drug interactions or use of medications that treat the same disease process.

CONTENTS

CHAPTER 1

Alpha Aα: Father

Tumeric, my heart bleeds for my father.

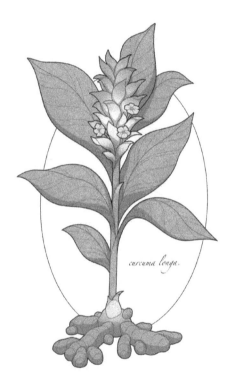

curcuma longa.

> Curcuma longa also known as Tumeric is effective against neuronal, cardiac, and kidney disorders.[1]

The Greek letter *alpha* means "arising, transcending, rising above." The concept of arising is the essence of divinity and immortality.

FATHER

When I was thirteen years old, a lot of unexpected changes occurred in my life that changed the direction of my life journey. My family elders used to say that nothing happens in life by chance. I have come to know that all the events that have occurred throughout my life have allowed me to have a greater understanding of my journey. Little did I know that I was about to start my experience with the end-of-life care, which became one of the most significant and rewarding experiences a person could ever imagine.

My parents separated when I was thirteen, and I was devastated. Fortunately, my father did not move far away. I would walk out my back door, cross the yard into the neighbor's yard, and literally be in my father's backyard. I was upset with my mother for a while because of the separation and because later, things changed in my household. I really didn't know why my parents separated; all I knew was that I loved them both. Most of all, I wanted them with me.

In the morning, my mother would put me on the school bus, and my father would meet me at the bus stop in the afternoon. But in the afternoon, my father had a real challenge. I was going through an adjustment to high school with new peers. Sometimes, those days were challenging—not to mention the competitiveness of every activity. I was oblivious to it all until the reality of understanding someone else's perception hit me in the face. I was learning how to manage and deal with girl groups, cliques, and bullies.

As the school bus got closer to my father's home each day, I could see my father standing there waiting for me at the bus stop. I knew he did not want me to be saddened by the events of the day, dealing with negative comments from peers, which came my way for several months. But I also knew that he understood I had to stand up for myself. My family was not the type to start discord, but we were not weak or cowardly, either.

My father, Robert Wright, was slim, with light, cinnamon-colored skin. His black hair was beginning to thin and change to salt and pepper.

He always wore suspenders—that was something men wore during the 1970s in rural Kentucky. My father was a strong, hardworking man. We lived on a farm before moving into town when he decided that it was his time to give up farming and retire. To me, my father's age was masked by his strength and determination.

His smile was warm and kind. His presence prevented me from allowing the events of the day to replay in my mind. Some days, when we were walking home, I noticed that my dad would walk a little slower.

As time went on, I adapted to my new living situation. On the weekends, I would wake up and have breakfast with my mother. Then I would take off out of her back door and skip over to my father's back door. Dad was always up and waiting for me. I wanted to check on him to make sure he was OK. I did not want him to be lonely since he lived alone, so I would come and go throughout the day, and sometimes we would have lunch together.

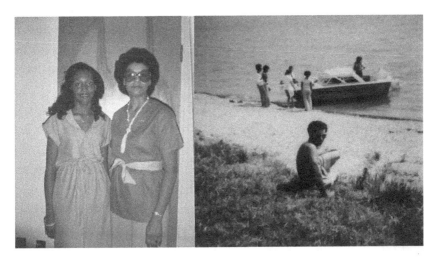

Most summers, I would leave the countryside and go stay with my sister—everyone calls her Pearl, but her real name is Laura—in the city for a week or two. She was so full of life, and family has always been most important to her. My visits with Laura and her family were always so much fun; she would take her son, daughter, and me to the local zoo and parks and on boat rides on the Belle of Louisville. I would ride a bicycle throughout the suburbs of Newburg with my niece, nephew, cousins, and friends. It was ironic that Pearl was the youngest girl before I was born, because being the matriarch seemed to suit her best. She still knows more family members than anyone in our family. She even has all their phone numbers and calls to remind them about family reunions (although they've been held on the same weekend ever since I was a child!).

Life was beginning to become normal for me again by early summer 1973, and I was happy. I went to visit with my brother George, who owned and lived on a dairy farm. He had this infectious laugh with a bright smile. He never met a stranger, and as a result, he was well known in the community. He was an active parent of fifteen children. Yes, I said *fifteen* children—eleven boys and four girls, all with the same wife.

George and his wife, Mary, were a team. They shared their home and love with everyone, but especially with extended family. I was always welcomed as an extended part of the immediate family. Their home was always immaculately kept; there were never any dirty dishes in the sink or clothes lying around the house. The washing machine and dryer seemed to run all day.

He took care of the farm and worked at General Electric to provide financially for the family. Mary made sure the household ran smoothly by canning, freezing, and storing the food produced on the farm. There were very few items ever purchased at the grocery store, other than bread. They both made sure education was a priority in their children's lives.

Their farm was about twenty-five minutes outside of town and off the main road. George and his family loved to go camping and boating and do many other outdoor activities. His sons George William and Larry would help drive to the campgrounds. If any of them became tired of driving, they never pulled off the road—they just switched drivers while driving. In those days, there was not a console between the seats, so they would literally stand up and switch drivers. Meanwhile, each person made sure that the other gripped the steering wheel while they changed positions. The van never swerved or wandered on the road. The first time I saw them do that, my mouth flew wide open and my heart pounded as I nervously looked for nearby cars and to see if we were staying on the road.

Mary would pull the boat when we drove to Green River. Most of their children could swim, but I could not. So I would put on a life vest and float around in the water until I drifted off farther than George's liking. Then he would swim out to me and bring me back closer to the boat.

One weekend, instead of camping, we went to King's Island Amusement Park. We left early that morning, and when we returned, everyone was just getting settled in bed when the phone rang. I overheard George from my niece's room upstairs because the phone he answered was near the staircase.

"Dad, if it is OK, I will bring her home first thing in the morning. I'm exhausted, and I don't feel safe driving right now. Is there anything wrong? OK, I promise I'll bring her home first thing in the morning."

I was excited to tell my dad about everything we did and saw at King's Island. But I wondered why he wanted me to come home, because I lived with my mother. I did not sleep well that night, mainly because of the anticipation of seeing my father the next day. When morning arrived, I got up, showered, dressed, and ate breakfast. Then I said goodbye to everyone and headed off to my mother's home with George.

On the way home, we laughed and talked about all the fun we'd had throughout the week. During the drive, I thought about how I planned to run in, drop my bags off, and then head straight over to dad's apartment to tell him all about my adventure.

When we arrived at my mother's house, I walked into the kitchen. I saw most of my family sitting there, including my brother Tommy, who at the time did not live there. My brother's eyes were red and almost closed. I could tell he had been crying. I asked, "What's wrong?"

My mother took me in her arms and said, "Your dad did not feel good last night, so he went to the hospital during the middle of the night. But he didn't make it. He died last night."

I looked at my mom in disbelief, and then I started out the back door, but Tommy grabbed me and pulled me back in the house.

George dropped his head and started shaking his head in sadness. In my thirteen-year-old mind, it seemed unreal. My father was strong. I could tell he was sad sometimes. I tried to make him happy, but I did not think his sadness should have caused him to die.

Mom said, "Your father had lung problems, and he was older."

I retaliated by saying, "You should not have made him go. We could have taken care of him, and he would still be here."

I broke loose from Tommy and sprinted outside to find my German Shepherd, Duke. I sat down, cried, and voiced all my thoughts to him. Duke was my furry friend. It seemed as though he understood everything I said, and over time, he helped heal my spirit from the devastating news. From then on, it seemed as though everything occurred in slow motion.

It started raining during the funeral-service procession. I later learned there's an old saying that if rain falls on a funeral procession, the deceased will go to heaven. Although many of my family members and friends were at the funeral, I could not bring myself to talk to anyone. I just stared off into space, trying to make sense of it all. All I could think was, *If only I had gone home that night, I could have kept my father alive.* As we walked behind his casket to the burial site, my shoes squished in the moist soil. I thought if I could just get stuck there in the mud, I wouldn't have to go to his grave site.

It was painful to let him go. I do not even remember if his casket was open during the service. I think I blocked it from my mind.

My mother, Juanita, was a full-figured woman shaped like a Coke bottle with long, black hair streaked with gray and mocha-colored skin. About a year after my father's death, my mother had a friend who would come over from time to time to fix broken things around the house. Sometimes, he would stay and play cards with my mother. I wanted nothing to do with him, even though he was always cordial to me. I was a smart little girl; I knew that he was only nice to me because he liked my mother.

She made sure we went to church every Sunday, unless someone was sick. Mother was a Eucharistic minister and sang in the church choir. People would walk by our house and yell, "Hello, Mrs. Juanita, so sorry to hear about Mr. Robert, or 'Doc.'" Our community was small, and most people knew each other or at least knew of someone who knew of each family. Whenever anyone discussed my dad, I would think to myself, *I hope Dad is OK.* I wanted to tell my mother that if she had not made Dad leave, he would still be there with us. I would have taken care of him. But I was raised not to talk back, so I would just leave the room to get away from the conversation.

I returned to school the week after his funeral. The competition started up again, but this time there was a diversion: I decided to join a dance group. The four of us in the group had attended parochial school together. We would practice several times a week after school. I decided to walk home from school one day after practice. I could have asked my mother to pick me up, but I needed the time to think. When I got home, my mother had a long conversation with me. I prayed to God to ask him for guidance and to take care of Daddy since I could not anymore.

God must have heard my prayers, because the adjustment period ended, and I soon graduated from high school. I was headed off to college to become a nurse. My mother was a nursing assistant at the local hospital. She often shared stories about her coworkers and events of her workday with us. Her stories about patients captivated me, and I knew I wanted to help others. I also realized that whether my father had lived with us or alone had no effect on his death. He was seventy-four years old and had been ill for many years. I also learned later that he had a history of clotting and cardiac disease. My mother's companion was still around, but now I found comfort in knowing that she would not be alone while I was away at school.

While in college, I met a young man who swept me off my feet, and later, we married. We started our family and were blessed with two children. One day while standing in the kitchen of our home, I cried and thought, *I wish my dad were here to see my children. He would really enjoy them.* In that instant, I felt a warmth around me as if I was receiving a hug. I thought with excitement, *Is that Dad?* No, it must've been wishful thinking. But it was summertime, and the air conditioner was on. The warmth was a feeling of comfort and not of heat. I had lost my Earthly father, but I never lost my heavenly father.

"Yet you, Lord, are our Father. We are the clay; you are the potter. We are all the work of your hand." (Isaiah 64:8, New International Version)

"Love is patient, love is kind. It does not envy, it does not boast, it is not proud.

It does not dishonor others, it is not self seeking, it is not easily angered, it keeps no record of wrongs. Love does not delight in evil but rejoices with the truth.

It always protects, always trusts, always hopes, always perseveres. Love never fails. But where there are prophecies, they will cease, where there are tongues, they will be stilled; where there is knowledge it will pass away. For we know in part and we prophesy in part, but when completeness comes, what is in our part disappears.

When I was a child, I talked like a child, I thought like a child, I reasoned like a child. When I became a man, I put the ways of childhood behind me. For now, I only see a reflection as in a mirror, then shall see face to face. Now I know in part, then I shall know full even as I am fully known. And these three remain, faith, hope, and love. But the greatest of these is love." (1 Corinthians 13:4–13, New International Version)

The first Bible verse acknowledges that God is my perfect heavenly father above all else. God molds us and can break us when necessary. The second Bible verse defines what love truly is in all relationships. Also, God wants us to understand that he expects us to grow and nurture our minds and our relationships, but especially the spiritual relationship we have with God.

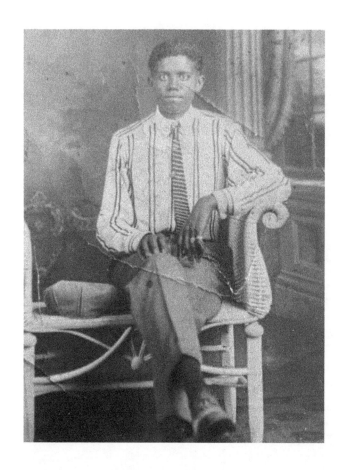

"Love is what motivates us all. We all desire unconditional love."

-My father, Robert Wright

CHAPTER 2

Beta Bβ: The Lesson

Like the juniperus communis, the lesson
inhibited my thoughts about cancer.

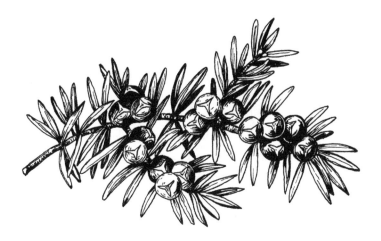

Juniperus communis suppressed cell growth in esophageal squamous cell carcinoma.[2]

The Greek letter *beta* means "basis," which is defined as "the bottom or base of anything, the part on which something stands or rests."

MRS. PERKINS

While I was in nursing school during the eighties, I decided to work at a local hospital to increase my exposure to the medical field. I secured a job as a nursing assistant in the Oncology Unit. At first, it seemed as though the requirements were pretty straightforward: taking vital signs; assisting patients with daily living activities such as bathing, brushing teeth, dressing, and eating; and completing tasks such as changing the linens on patients' beds when necessary to help keep them comfortable.

These are simple things we do on a daily basis but sometimes take for granted; we think we will always be able to perform these tasks independently. In reality, for some people, there may be a period in their lives when they need assistance. Mrs. Perkins, a patient in that unit, troubled my mind. She was dying of esophageal cancer; due to its location, it was inoperable. The left side of her neck was black, which is called *eschar*. The tumor protruded outward at least two inches beyond the normal circumference of her neck. The rest of her skin was creamy white, with some discolorations.

It was difficult for me to see how invasive the tumor was. Even at rest, her breathing was slightly labored. She did not speak, open her eyes, or make any type of communication other than a slight moan when she was being repositioned. I usually notified the nurse when I was going to move her, just in case it was time to medicate her for pain. To my knowledge, Mrs. Perkins never had any visitors. I found myself making rounds more frequently at her bedside, since she could not communicate her needs.

After several days, she started perspiring profusely, which required frequent linen changes. I realized her perspiration was due to her heavy breathing, despite oxygen being provided by high-flow nasal cannula. I used washcloths to keep the moisture off her face. At a minimum, her sheets were changed at least twice a shift in addition to changing her body's position every two hours to prevent pressure ulcers. I was so tired after my shift, but at the same time, I wanted to do more to help ease her discomfort. At least I could keep her dry, which I hoped provided her some comfort. The next day when I returned, her breathing was even more laborious. The nurse medicated her, but that time, it was not effective. The doctor ordered bilevel positive airway pressure, or BiPap. The advantage to this machine is that it is noninvasive. That means medical staff aren't required to insert an endotracheal tube for mechanical ventilation—instead, a patient wears a face mask or nasal plugs that forces air into the lungs.

An ET tube is a specific tube inserted into the mouth to establish and maintain an open airway for exchange of carbon dioxide and oxygen. With BiPap, the physician orders a specific rate of respirations or breaths per minute. I stood there watching, expecting to see some relief for her. I felt as though I could barely keep up with the frequency of linen changes. The increased workload from breathing increased the cardiac workload. So, for the previous two days, this woman had probably felt like she had run a marathon, but rest had finally come. She stopped breathing, and her heartbeat ceased. I wondered if the growth of that tumor restricted her airway at that point, or if her heart had just given up.

Visions of her suffering would remain ingrained in my memory as long as the stars will remain in our sky. That memory of her blocked every thought of me ever wanting treatment for cancer if I were to ever receive that diagnosis. It seemed as though she had no relief from her discomfort.

I know now that there are many modalities of treatment, such as homeopathic interventions like juniperus communis. The course of treatment for pain management is also different today. During the 1980s, inadequate pain management for oncology patients was under review by health-care providers, according to the *Cancer Journal Clinical* published on March 30, 2018. Based on the information reviewed by the authors of this document, their research determined that, "poor communication between the patient and providers was an essential variable contributing to health-related quality of life."

The goal was to effectively manage cancer-related pain without putting a patient at risk of opioid addiction. The presence and severity of pain, as well as other pain-management modalities, should be individually based on quality-of-life or end-of-life pain management. It is imperative to focus on managing pain or discomfort during the end-of-life process, including frequent monitoring of patients' conditions, especially if they cannot verbalize their needs. Continually educating new clinicians is vital to helping them determine the difference between medication tolerance, addiction, and substance disorder and appropriately assess and relay vital information to the physician so that pain of any type can be adequately managed.

> "Blessed be God, even the Father of our Lord Jesus Christ, The Father of mercies, and the God of all comfort; Who comforteth us in all our tribulation, that we may be able to comfort them which are in any trouble, by the comfort wherewith we ourselves are comforted of God. For as the suffering of Christ abound in us, so our consolation and salvation, which is effectual in the enduring of the same sufferings which we also suffer; or whether we be comforted, it is for your consolations and salvation. And our hope of you is steadfast, knowing, that as ye are partaker of the sufferings, so shall ye be also of the consolation." (2 Corinthians 1:3–7, King James Version)

> "Likewise, the Spirit also helps in our weakness. For we do not know what we should pray for as we ought: but the Spirit itself maketh intercession for us with groaning which cannot be uttered." (Romans 8:26, King James Version)

These two Bible verses remind me that God is our comforter and protector. God uses people to help us when we cannot speak on our own behalf. Nurses advocate for their patients, especially when they are their most vulnerable.

When I graduated from nursing school, a friend gave me a bookmark with this nurse's prayer on it, by Robin Eagle. The prayer for nurses was new to me; I don't think either of us had any idea how many times I would read it.

THE NURSE'S PRAYER

"May I be a nurse, Lord, with gentle healing hands,
who always speaks with kindness,
who cares, and understands.
And while I'm serving others as you would have me to do.
Please help me remember that I am truly serving you."

CHAPTER 3

Epsilon Eε: Reality

*Fireweed is an astringent that might have
been beneficial to Mrs. Smith.*

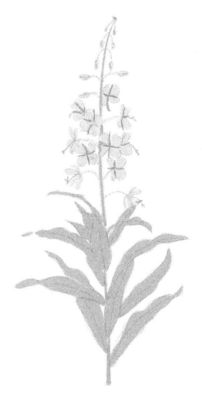

Fireweed is used to treat pain and swelling, fevers, tumors, and wounds. It is also used as an astringent and a tonic.[3]

The Greek letter *epsilon* means "essence," which is defined as "the basic, real, and invariable nature of a thing or its significant individual feature."

MRS. SMITH

Mrs. Smith was fifty-nine years old with altered mental status related to a urinary tract infection. When she first arrived, she was pleasant but confused.

She would say, "I was just thinking about what our president is going to do about his economy. You know those Kennedys always come up with a plan."

But it was 1997, and Kennedy was not our president. I never challenged her subject matter; I just went along with the conversation. Becoming confrontational with her would serve no purpose. It would have only agitated her more and caused all of us more grief. As a health-care provider, you must learn to pick your battles.

She was receiving intravenous fluids because, despite our best efforts, she could not consume enough fluids to improve her hydration status. I noticed a cold sore starting to erupt on her lower lip, so I called her primary doctor to inform him. He ordered a consultation with a dermatologist. I called the dermatologist on call to let him know of the new order. When I returned to work, I noticed during my first rounds that Mrs. Smith looked weaker and even more fragile than when she had first arrived. I thought her mentation would have improved by the time I returned.

I read what the dermatologist had determined from his consultation. He had written an order recommending Zovirax by mouth for the cold sore. I checked the old medication orders, but there was no order for the medication anywhere on the medication record. I called the primary doctor to inform him of that and the lack of improvement in her mentation. He ordered the medication, per the consulting doctor's recommendations. Since he was already on the premises, I also asked him if he would come evaluate the patient because of her increased confusion.

He said, "I am busy in the emergency room. I will come up when I get a chance."

I thought, *Why don't you just come up to check her out and then go back down and complete what you are doing there?*

The respiratory therapist, Phil, was on the floor to evaluate and administer Mrs. Smith's inhaler. He pointed behind her head and asked, "What caused this change? This is different from yesterday."

"I can only imagine," I responded. "I am working on that now. She had some diarrhea before you arrived. She was getting IV fluids a few days ago, but that order was stopped. I think I am going to put an IV in her because this is a change since I was last here."

Phil said, "I am going to stay here while you do that because I think you are going to need me."

She was so dehydrated that I could only get a #24 IV in; a #24 gauge is a small opening, but it was better than nothing. Then I went out to the nurse's station to call the doctor again. Barbara said, "What is going on? You look frustrated."

"I am trying to get the doctor to come to the floor to evaluate Mrs. Smith, but he keeps putting me off. I need him to come up here."

I called the doctor again to provide an update on my findings and her recent vital signs.

"Hello, Dr. Truitt, I wanted to let you know that Mrs. Smith is more lethargic, and her vital signs are T 98.3; P 104; R 16; BP 98/60. The respiratory therapist is here giving her an inhaler, and she cannot inhale, so he is going to give her a neb treatment. Also, her confusion is increasing. Can we order some labs on her and possibly some IV fluids? I really think you need to come see her."

Dr. Truitt sighed deeply and then replied, "OK. Order her a CMP and CBC, and start NS at a hundred ccs per hour. I will be up when I can."

We had just changed shifts, and it is common practice for clinicians to evaluate the critical patients first.

I called the phlebotomist to notify her of the order and gathered the IV fluids and tubing. When I arrived at Mrs. Smith's bedside, Sherry, a seasoned phlebotomist, was present. She attempted to draw her blood but was unsuccessful.

She said, "I can't get anything from her. Can I draw some blood from your IV?"

"Ok, only if you go slow, so you don't blow the vein." I hung the fluids on the pole, started opening the clamp on the tubing, and adjusted the infusion pump, per the order. Mrs. Smith's body became limp. I rubbed her arm, called her name, and did a sternal rub on her chest, but she was unresponsive.

I punched the "Code Blue" button in the room. Phil connected the Ambu bag to supply oxygen, and I performed chest compressions. The charge nurse arrived with the code cart, and she started noting information. Once the code team arrived, I got out of the way and went to call Dr. Truitt to inform him of the code blue.

He arrived on the floor and said, "What happened?"

I was even more frustrated with his comment. "What do you mean? In between which phone call do you need me to fill you in?"

You could have heard a pin drop in that room. The only sound was coming from the Ambu bag being squeezed. I gathered my thoughts and then started explaining, because it would not benefit the patient if I did not supply the important information that had led up to that event. The emergency-room doctor attempted to insert a triple-lumen catheter. This type of catheter is preferred because it has three infusion channels, but he was unsuccessful in the internal jugular. He then attempted to insert a line in the groin into the femoral vein, without success.

He said to me, "I can't believe you got an IV in her. She is so dry." She was so dehydrated that it was difficult to thread the cannula into the vein.

After many minutes, the physician called an end to our efforts, and the time of death was pronounced. I wanted to cry. I was a new nurse; I wanted to save everyone.

When I returned to the room to clean up, it looked like there had been an explosion of medical equipment; it was scattered all around the room from our efforts. I began by removing all the sharp items. I saw three used central-line kits from the physician's desperate efforts to find a viable vein.

I learned from that experience just how quickly a patient's status can change, as well as the importance of communicating reports from consulted providers to the primary physician. At that time, we used paper charts instead of computers to communicate patient information. (Yes, I am from the dinosaur era.) I also learned that despite all our efforts, there are some people who we are unable to be saved—and that was the hardest lesson.

Fireweed is a natural astringent that can be used to heal cold sores.

> "Do not be anxious about anything, but in everything by prayer and supplication with thanksgiving let your request be made know to God." (Philippians 4:6-7, English Standard Version)

> "We love him, because he first loved us." (1 John 4:19, King James Version)

These Bible verses remind me of God's love for us. We must turn our worry and stress over to God and then let it go. God's peace will guard our hearts and mind.

CHAPTER 4

Gamma Γγ: Arousing the Spirit

*Mrs. Goveart clarifies my thoughts like
bur marigold clarifies the kidneys.*

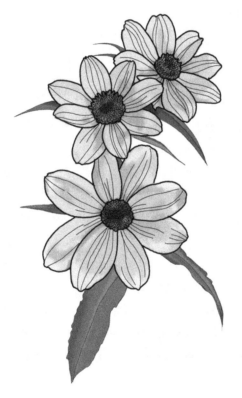

Bur marigold is used to treat urinary tract infections, the kidney, and respiratory ailments.[4]

Gamma is the Greek letter that means "generative and creative." The shape of the letter, *Γ*, suggests an offshoot from a stem, a sprout.

MRS. GOVEART

It was 6:40 p.m. on the fourth floor of the hospital, and everyone was arriving and getting ready for the shift report. Three staff members were working that night: April, the charge nurse; Barbara, the nursing tech; and me, a staff nurse. Our census was twelve patients. I heard April talking as I walked into the break room.

"Hey, Barbara; how are you doing?"

"OK. I am just coming from my grandson's football practice," Barbara replied.

"Oh, what position will he be playing on the team?" April asked.

"Running back."

"Wow! I am sure you are proud of him," April said.

"We will talk more later. I'm going to get the report," said Barbara.

April then turned and handed me the census and stated, "Tonight should be a good night. We have six patients apiece, and they seem to be stable. Bernice, you take the last six, and I'll take the first six. Mrs. Goveart is due for peritoneal dialysis tonight. Have you done that with her? She has a routine that works for her, and she doesn't like to deviate from it."

"Yes, I have. She is so proficient at doing it. I teased her about getting a job here specializing in peritoneal dialysis. She is such a kind lady," I replied.

After the report, I visited Mrs. Goveart first to notify her what time we would start her dialysis. She was the most unstable patient I would provide care for that night. As I walked in her room, I was greeted by her sweet-tempered voice.

"Hi, Bernice. I was wondering if you were going to be here tonight. You know I worry about my daughter, Vikki. She does not have any children to keep her busy, but Debbie has a husband and children."

"From what I have seen, you have two loving daughters who care a lot about you and each other. I will be back shortly. Is there anything I can get for you before I leave? Barbara will be in shortly to check on your vital signs, and she will bring you a snack if you would like one."

"No. I know you will be back, and if I need you, I will call," Mrs. Goveart replied.

I continued my rounds. As I walked down the hallway to my next patient's room, Mr. Jones, I spotted Barbara and decided to give her a report.

"Hey, Barbara; I want to update you on our patients."

"OK, Bernice. Hang on; I'm coming." Barbara dropped off water to a patient's room and then returned to the hallway.

"So, we have Mrs. Goveart, seventy-one, with peritoneal dialysis, which is due tonight. She has been performing the dialysis at home but became febrile and is here for antibiotics. She ambulates independently, full code, alert, and oriented times four. Make sure you keep strict track of her intake and output. Mr. Jones, a sixty-eight-year-old male who is three days post-op of a right hip replacement by Dr. Brown. His wound has been draining a lot. So check his bandage to make sure it is not getting saturated while making rounds. Also check his bed alarm to make sure it is on, hip precautions, ambulates with a walker, and a full code. Mrs. Michael, sixty-four, is here for exacerbation of COPD, and she never sleeps in the bed. Make sure you keep her feet elevated because of the edema, full code, and 1500 fluid restriction."

"Is she continent?" Barbara asked.

"Yes, she uses the bedside commode, but if she has a coughing spell, she is incontinent, so check her brief. She is on four liters of oxygen via nasal cannula. Then we have Mrs. Thompson, fifty-nine. She is here with altered mental status related to dehydration and urinary tract infection. She's more alert during the day, so make sure you have her alarms on as well. She is a full code. Mr. Santos, sixty-two, just had an ACD placement. He was transferred from another hospital. He is stable and here for physical therapy. If he complains of dizziness or shortness of breath, let me know as soon as possible. He is on room air now, but we know that can change. He is a 'do not resuscitate.'

"Then we have Mr. Johnson, sixty-seven, here with gout and uncontrolled diabetes mellitus type two. Make sure you check his glucometer before you give him a snack. Ambulates independently, full code. Let me know if anyone's vital signs are out of range and if you need help."

I made my way back to Mrs. Goveart's room after everyone had been given their medications for the night. "Hey, Mrs. Goveart, sorry to keep you waiting."

"No problem. I was just sitting here thinking about Vikki and Debbie."

I set things up in the room to prepare for dialysis while Mrs. Goveart talked.

"Debbie's children will keep her and her husband busy. Vikki's husband is very supportive of her, and I know she will be in good hands. He is very good to her, but his job requirements are time sensitive. He is very busy, which gives her more time to focus on me. She treats me like I am her child. She worries about me all the time. They both always make sure I have everything I need."

"It seems as though you are blessed to have such a wonderful family. How are you feeling? We're almost done," I replied.

"I'm a little tired. I had a busy day," said Mrs. Goveart.

"I am sure you are tired. The physical therapists provide extensive therapy because they want to make sure you are safe and able to function independently before you go home. I am going to disconnect you now." I paused and looked in her eyes. "If you would like to talk more, just call me.

"I'm glad you are here; thank you. I'm sure you have lots of paperwork to do. I'm going to go to sleep for now. I'll see you in the morning," she said.

During rounds, we observed Mrs. Goveart sleep throughout the night. In the morning, I saw her wave at me as she walked toward the bathroom door. After the report, I walked down the hall to Mrs. Goveart's room and knocked at the door.

"Hi, Mrs. Goveart. I have something I would like to give you. If you are uncomfortable with this and would prefer not to take it, I understand."

I extended my hand out to show her the medal. Saint Philomena has always given me comfort whenever I have a lot on my mind.

"I would like to give this medal to you and say a prayer, if that is OK."

"Oh, I would really appreciate that," said Mrs. Goveart.

SAINT PHILOMENA PRAYER

Hail, O Saint Philomena, Virgin and Martyr
Patroness of the children of Mary whom
God glorifies by so many miracles,
We rely on your aid.
Obtain for us the grace to be faithful To Jesus Christ even to death.

Three days later, I returned to work.

"Hey, Bernice, you took care of Mrs. Goveart the last time we worked, right? Well, the charge nurse just told me that she was refusing dialysis because her labs have not improved. She is tired, and her family is at her bedside. She changed her code status from full code to do not resuscitate," said April.

Oh no; she had been so strong during this hospitalization. I hoped she would reconsider, but I knew I had to respect her decision. During rounds, as I was checking on Mrs. Goveart, I saw her daughter standing outside the door of her room with her head down. I approached Vikki.

"Hi. How are you doing?"

Vikki started to cry as she embraced me. "She has always had faith. She acknowledges there is a spirit higher than herself. My mother is the sweetest person I know. I am really going to have a hard time with losing her," she said.

"I am sure you will, but I know she would want you to persevere. She has so much respect and love for you both, but you have a special place in her heart."

"I know she worries because I don't have any children. She also feels her death will be harder for me. I know that we have been lucky to have her here as long as we have. She is right—I will miss her more than Debbie will, only because I tend to spend more time with her. I don't have as many responsibilities as Debbie. I think I am going to spend the night. She seems a lot weaker to me. I think Debbie is going to stay also," said Vikki.

"OK, I will get some chairs and linens for you both later. I want to check on her first."

I entered the room, where Mrs. Goveart was resting in the bed with her daughter, Debbie, at her bedside. Debbie's husband was seated in the chair near her bed.

Mrs. Goveart said, "Hi, Bernice. You've been off for a few days. I missed you. I am glad you are here tonight."

"So am I. You decided to stop the dialysis."

"Yes. I am just getting worse. It is time for me."

Mrs. Goveart looked down. I sighed; I understood what she was trying to say. I repositioned her for comfort. She reached her hand out, and I held it until she relaxed. I noticed that the medal I had given her was pinned to her gown. That gave me some hope that she had received comfort from the prayer I had said with her.

During my rounds, I went into her room periodically throughout the night. Debbie came out of the room for a beverage, which gave us a chance to talk.

"Mom would attend Sunday services with me faithfully before she started her dialysis treatments. She enjoyed reading her Bible frequently, if not daily, and she believes in Jesus. I know she has a personal relationship with him, and she has accepted his gift of salvation during church services. Mom saw to it that Vikki and I went to Sunday school and church from elementary through our high school years. She taught us the Christian children's bedtime prayer and the Lord's Prayer. She prayed with us each night until we were old enough to pray on our own," said Debbie.

"How blessed you are to have such a wonderful mother who taught you both about spirituality. Not everyone can say that."

During the next round, the lighting was dimmed in her room to promote rest. The family had been at her side for several hours.

Mrs. Goveart awoke as I entered the room and said, "I have all three."

Her son-in-law said, "The Father, Son, and Holy Spirit."

She said, "Yesssss," and then nodded and smiled with so much joy and peace. Then she said, "All these people keep coming up to me who I don't know."

Her son-in-law said, "She is seeing angels."

We all smiled and nodded. As I was repositioning her, she opened her eyes, grabbed my hand, and said, "It is your father!"

I gasped and tears came to my eyes, but I held them back. I excused myself. As I closed the door, tears flooded my face. Barbara and April were standing in the hallway and approached me.

April asked, "Oh, did she pass?"

I said no as I wiped tears away. "I have had many conversations with her, but I have never mentioned anything about my father. My father is dead. So how could she have known to say that she was seeing my father, if he was not there?"

They both looked at me and gasped. "What?" they said in unison.

I just started crying again.

"You should go take a break. I will check on them," said April.

I went to the break room and just sat there, trying to make sense out of what just happened. *But why is he here? He must want me to know something.*

I reflected back on the day many years ago when I had felt warmth while standing in my kitchen, crying. I thought, *I wish my father could have seen them.* I started walking up the hallway, but then I thought, *I better go back to check on Mrs. Goveart.* When I opened the door, I could see extensive mottling on her body, but amazingly, she was still talking to her family! Wow, how could this be? I dared not turn any lights on because I thought the sight of her would frighten her family. To be honest, it unnerved me a little. I left the room but stood outside the door.

I felt like I needed to go back into her room. I opened the door slowly, and I could see her lifeless body.

Mrs. Goveart was a very special person. God had allowed her to share her experience with us right up until she departed this Earth.

After her daughters left the nursing unit, I performed her postmortem care with Barbara. I stood there submerged in my thoughts of what had just occurred. I was unaware whether her daughters realized that my father was one of the strange people she had seen. If there was ever a doubt in my mind about God, after what I had just experienced, they were gone.

For weeks, I thought about what had happened. It was an amazing experience that I would never forget—nor would I ever forget Mrs. Goveart. She had opened my eyes to realize that there is eternal life. My father and I were very close, and I believe he wanted me to know that he has been right by my side all this time. I realized that Mrs. Goveart was trying to tell me from the beginning of my shift that she was waiting for me to be there because of the relationship I had formed with her daughters and her. Several months after her death, I received a letter from Debbie and Vikki, to my surprise. I wondered how they had found my address, but I was really grateful they had. I felt as though receiving their letters was a confirmation on how truly wonderful that experience was. My experience with Mrs. Goveart sprouted and created new thoughts about end-of-life care.

Dear Bernice,

You'll never know how much Vikki and I appreciated all you did for our mom, Beverly Foxcart, during her stay in the Transitional Care Unit last fall. We are sincerely grateful for the care and concern you gave Mom, especially as the end was drawing near for her. The way you stood by her and us until she drew her last breath, meant so much to us and impressed us deeply. Your hugs and gentle manner gave us a great amount of comfort.

Mom had a beautiful funeral service. She wore the St. Philomena medal you gave her, but I kept it as a reminder of the comfort you provided to my sister and me during the most sorrowful time in our personal lives.

Thank you for everything, Bernice you are a very special person and a wonderful nurse. We'll never forget you.

Love, Debbie

"Blessed are the pure in heart, for they shall see God."
(Matthew 5:8, New King James Version)

"Who hath saved us, and called us with an holy calling,
not according to our works, but according to his own
purpose and grace, which was given us in Christ Jesus
before the world began." (2 Timothy 1:9, King James
Version)

The first Bible verse acknowledges that if you are able to maintain
the ritual laws of God and are pure in your devotion to God, you will
see him. To me, the second Bible verse acknowledges that we all have a
purpose through God's grace, which was bestowed upon us before we
were even born.

CHAPTER 5

Zeta Zξ: Medication versus the human spirit

Like sage reduces stress, Mr. Winkler teaches us what not to stress about.

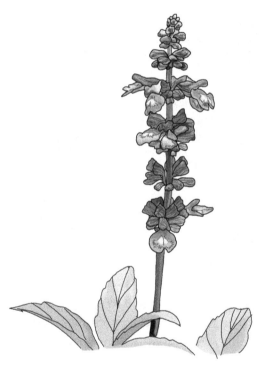

Sage relieves sore throat pain, reduces oxidative stress in the body, increases calmness counteracting depression, and improves mood.[5]

The letter *Z*, the symbol of the Greek letter *zeta*, means "spark of life."

MR. WINKLER

Mr. Winkler, a sixty-eight-year-old male, was admitted with failure to thrive related to metastatic cancer. He was a six-foot-tall, frail, emaciated-appearing man. When he first came to the unit, he had a trachea tube in place related to esophageal cancer. He could communicate with us through gestures and with the use of a communication chart.

Mr. Winkler's PICC line—a peripherally inserted central catheter that can stay in longer and reduce the number of needle sticks needed—was in place for him to receive morphine for pain management. It seemed as though every day, we were increasing his dosage and providing a bolus, or a one-time extra dose, for management of his pain. During rounds, he would point at the communication board or Wong-Baker FACES pain-rating scale and indicate that his pain was either an eight or nine out of ten, which indicated severe to worst pain. His body language indicated pain—he grimaced, frequently moved in the bed, and walked guardedly from the bed to the chair.

His family members were surprised to see how much weight he had lost related to the cancer. But we were surprised at how agile he was, considering the amount of medication he had received and his decrease in appetite. He was refusing all assistive devices, such as an indwelling catheter and feeding tube. I asked the family if there was someone he might want to visit that had not seen him yet.

His sister said, "Yes, our brother has not come in yet. He works in Virginia during the week. He should be able to come in this weekend. I know he is not doing well. The doctor told him that it is only a matter of time. I am really surprised to see him up and about. He has lost so much weight. It pains me to think of what he must be feeling."

I thanked her for the update.

"Yes, we think that he is hanging on to see him. I have to leave now, but I will be back this weekend."

The telephone started ringing at the nurses' station.

"OK, let me know if there is anything else you think of that we can do to help," I said and walked over to answer the phone. "Level four Bernice; how can I help you?"

"Hi, this is Phil, the pharmacist. I was just calling to check on the patient in 416. He has been getting that seventy-five milligram of morphine for several days now. I just wanted to be sure it is not leaking out into the bed."

At that time, seventy-five milligrams per hour was a lethal dose. While I was talking to the pharmacist, I could hear Becky's voice and the sound of Mr. Winkler's side rails moving.

"Bernice, I need you now!" Becky called.

"Oh no, I have to go. I will call you back later." I hung up the phone and sprinted toward his room.

As I approached the door, I saw Becky struggling with Mr. Winkler; his arms and legs were moving. Then I saw Becky fall backward against the wall from his force. I soon realized that she had been trying to keep him from removing the trach's inner cannula because suddenly, I saw a silver piece flying through the air. After assisting Becky, I picked up the inner cannula and walked out of the room to call the doctor to let him know what had just happened. Mr. Winkler sat up in bed and watched as Becky and I walked out the door.

"Dr. Smith, this is Bernice. I just want to let you know that Mr. Winkler just pulled out his trach."

Dr. Smith said, "Is he breathing OK? If he doesn't want it in, just leave it out. That must be what he wants. I am sure his stoma will stay open. He has had that trach for a long time."

I monitored his trach site frequently, but it never closed. The trach had been in so long that his skin remained dilated. Thank goodness for that!

Becky giggled and said, "I'm not hurt physically, but my pride might be bruised a little."

We laughed and joked about that for a few minutes. You have to find some humor in the midst of it all. I was glad that was the only trauma she had experienced.

We continued to monitor the severity and frequency of his pain, which continued to increase, which meant more medication boluses. He was still restless and frequently attempted to get out of the bed without assistance. We were concerned that he might fall.

On Saturday, his brother arrived. He sat with Mr. Winkler. For the first time since his admission, Mr. Winkler sat in bed, nodding, and appeared to be relaxed. He reached his hand out for his brother's hand, and they both nodded again. I hoped this was the person he had been waiting for. Maybe now he could have some peace. His brother sat at his bedside for probably two hours.

He seemed peaceful, but toward the end of his brother's visit, his troubled demeanor resurfaced. After his brother left, his cousin called him. This was when the change began. His posture became more relaxed. He did not request breakthrough pain medications. He no longer attempted to get out of bed without assistance. Mr. Winkler had completed all the tasks he needed in order to have peace. That old saying, "Peace comes from within," now had new meaning and reverence with me. By morning, Mr. Winkler's spirit had left for us to perform postmortem care on his body. His body remained for his family to acknowledge the end of his journey on Earth.

Optimal Pain Management for Patients with Cancer in the Modern Era, an article written by, Bethann Scarborough, MD, and Cardinale B. Smith, MD, PhD. Defines understanding pharmacology for opioid management requires identification of the three primary opioid receptors within the body—the mu, kappa, and delta receptors; genetic variations in receptors are one factor contributing to the varying response to opioids within or between individuals. An exception is transmucosal route immediate release fentanyl, aka fentanyl pop, which releases within sixty to ninety minutes. This method offers several advantages over traditional metabolism by the liver.

Of course, most patients who require end-of-life care might not have normal liver or kidney function.

Mr. Winkler's experience sparked new ways of thinking about pain management for oncology patients for me.

"And I heard a voice from heaven saying, write this: Blessed are the dead who die in the Lord from now on. Blessed indeed, says the Spirit, that they may rest from their labors, for their deeds follow them!" (Revelations 14:13, King James Version)

"But rejoice, inasmuch as ye are partakers of Christ's sufferings; that, when his glory shall be revealed, ye may be glad also with exceeding joy." (1 Peter 4:13, King James Version)

The first Bible verse speaks about the labor of both the body and soul—the labor of disease, inward troubles, doubts, and fears. All of us are going to die, but it is a privilege for believers, because the sting of death is removed by Christ. Mr. Winkler was literally emaciated, but his will was strong. God allowed him to persevere until his task was done. The second Bible verse acknowledges that providing care to anyone who is suffering is a difficult journey that is well worth the effort. Family members and medical staff suffer emotionally and physically while providing care because we are invested in the best interest of the patient. However, along the journey, our character and strength grow.

I heard this message during one Sunday church sermon:

"What I have learned is that death is just a pass from this life to our true life. The human body is inclined to death and sin. Sin is like an imprisonment of the body. In this life, we know, we must act to preserve and secure our everlasting life. For those of you that fear God, you know that by our sins we decide our own salvation or condemnation. Faith is worth a good fight, make the right choice each day. Faith is what we lean on. Stay awake because the devil is like a roaring lion looking for someone's faith to devour. Our words are taken by the wind and used against us. Facts and action are how we give our testimony. God loves us all the same. It is just up to us to let him in our lives."

CHAPTER 6

Eta Hη: The Spirit is Calling

Feeling as though Mullein could have saved me from the stars.

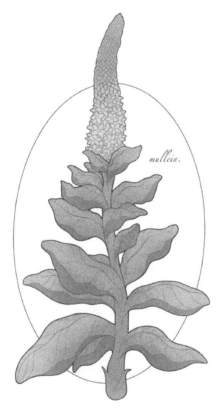

mullein.

Common mullein has been used to treat pulmonary problems, asthma, spasmodic coughs, migraine headaches, and inflammatory diseases.[6]

The Greek letter *eta* means "shared center," or "the turning point." Eta Carinae consists of two binary stars orbiting around each other, potentially due to winds and partial eclipses. I also had two children who circled around me all the time.

BERNICE

Many years ago, I didn't understand stress and its impact on our health. During one period in my life, I felt more stress. As a result of the stress, I developed asthma. I was already genetically predisposed to it, but the disease waited until later in my life to develop. It started as allergic symptoms that would trigger asthma attacks. I was constantly on steroids, and eventually, my doctor started implying that these symptoms were related to stress.

"What is causing your stress?" he would ask. How could I say, "My husband and life?" All couples go through a season of change, and that was our moment.

Southern women are taught to be strong and not to show weakness. But the truth was that communication was difficult for my husband, Arthur, and I at times. Back then, neither one of us was very effective at communicating our needs to each other. Instead, we avoided important conversations. Also, trying to adjust to a new community after moving from another state complicated matters even more. It took time to develop and nurture friendships with people within the community.

I had grown accustomed to receiving warm Southern hospitality. I had lived in several other states before we moved, and each time, we were greeted with a warm welcome. The ladies would make it a day of adventure by arriving at my front door and driving my daughter and me around, pointing out where the local grocery stores and malls were located. Instead, after this move, I met people who were polite but busy with their own lives. In my new surroundings, if you were an outsider, you remained at arm's length, which isolated you even further from the community.

There is always an exception, and there was one particular family that ran their own septic-tank business. They were community oriented and hosted an annual cookout that people from both inside and outside the county attended. It was probably one of the largest events in this community. Fortunately for me, there were other transplants into this community, and we formed our own support and family system.

One day, I had decided that this county, along with other stressors, was too much for me, and I was going to leave the state. That day and night, I was using my nebulizer every four hours. My asthma was out of control. I called my doctor's office early that morning. I was fortunate to get an early-morning appointment. Once I was at the doctor's office, I was seen by a new associate because my attending was not there. That doctor was not familiar with my history of asthma. She gave me a single dose of Solumedrol, which is a steroid injection. I asked her if she planned to start me on a tapering dose of steroids.

She said, "You should be fine with just the shot."

I replied, "Don't you think I might have a rebound reaction?" (That means the symptoms increase or worsen in severity once the injection wears off.)

She said, "No, you should be fine."

Fatigued from being up all night, I just went home and got into my bed. I could finally sleep because the frequent coughing spasms and mucus production had decreased. I awakened to the sound of my children coming through the door. I realized I needed to get up and start cooking dinner. This was around four in the afternoon. Around that same time, my husband arrived home.

"Hey Bernice, did you go to the doctor today?"

"Yes, they gave me a shot but no pills to take. I do feel a little better, but I am still tired."

I served dinner and was sitting at the table getting ready to eat when suddenly, I felt as though I could not get any air in my lungs. *OK*, I thought, *it's time for another nebulizer treatment.* I went upstairs and started using my nebulizer machine, but this time, it was not helping at all. I began to feel a little hot, so I turned on the ceiling fan. At that moment, my daughter came to check on me.

She said loudly, "Mom, are you all right?"

I could tell she could see a change in me. I tried to speak, but no words would come out. I felt like crying. I attempted again to speak, but nothing was coming out.

My daughter said, "You aren't breathing, are you? You just keep using your nebulizer. I am going to call 911." I could hear Jessica calling on the phone in the other room. My husband entered the room.

"Is that thing, the nebulizer not working?"

I heard the panic in his voice. I sat on the edge of the bed and sensed a weakness in myself, but I did not want to let on how bad I really felt. I thought I would be OK once the medic arrived, because they could give medications. Thank goodness I lived near an ambulance company, so it did not take long for them to arrive. The two male EMTs entered my bedroom. I was sitting on the bed, still attempting to obtain relief by using the nebulizer. I was on my second treatment when one of the EMTs started to examine me. My skin was clammy, and I could not speak. I didn't even want to know what my pulse oximetry was. I could tell by the looks on their faces that I was in trouble. I wanted to try to walk down the stairs; they said no and brought in a chair stretcher to carry me down. They took my vital signs and then swiftly carried me off on the stretcher after they inquired about the details before the attack. Thank God for Jessica; she relayed all the necessary information about my health history.

My husband was in shock; I could see the panic on his face. He kept asking the EMTs questions, and they kept repeating to him that I needed to go to the hospital. They were aware of the urgency of my condition. When we were outside the house, I was transferred to the stretcher. My husband tried to get into the ambulance with me. The EMT informed him that it was against the law for him to ride in the ambulance. Arthur looked at me as though he feared the worst.

Finally, one of the EMTs said, "You have to be able to drive yourself back home."

He understood that and got into his truck and began to follow the ambulance. My neighbor called to check on my children and offered to have them stay with her until my husband returned.

My daughter said, "We need to be home in case they call back. Thank you, but they won't know where we are."

En route to the hospital, the medic met the ambulance and inserted an IV and administered medication. I heard the ambulance driver radio the hospital.

"We have a priority one in route."

He went on to describe my symptoms and vital signs. I could hear the ambulance sirens blaring and I felt the cab moving, so I knew the driver was moving fast, and I was grateful. Oxygen was already in use with a nebulizer treatment. My clothes were beginning to dampen, and I realized I was in deep trouble. I just kept telling myself, *You will be all right once you get to the hospital.* This was not my first trip to the hospital for an asthma attack, but the attacks had never been this severe.

When I arrived at the hospital, as the stretcher turned the corner, the first person I saw was my friend Rachel, who is a respiratory therapist. She had worked the night shift for several years, and she was usually assigned to my unit. I thought, *Thank God; everything is going to be all right.* One night at work, we had discussed intubation and how patients fared afterwards. I had told her not to let anyone intubate me. I knew that I would be anxious because the tube for intubation is narrow. I told her if I passed out or if I was not making any sense, then to go for it, but otherwise to try to let the medication work. She had agreed.

When Rachel saw me, she said, "Bernice, what is going on?"

I could not speak, but she could read my lips.

I mouthed, "I'm glad you are here."

She looked worried as she connected me to the nebulizer. My breathing remained restricted, which increased the workload on my entire body. I could hear the doctor telling Rachel she was going to intubate me. At that time, it was protocol to intubate patients who did not respond to aggressive nebulizer treatments and a single dose of intravenous corticosteroids. I heard Rachel speaking on my behalf. She went round and round with the doctor. Thank goodness I never lost consciousness. For some reason, I began to smell a wonderful scent. I kept trying to figure out where it was coming from, so I got up and walked toward the bathroom, because it appeared to be stronger there.

Arthur said, "Why do you keep getting up? Every time you get up, your oxygen saturations drop! Stay in bed."

I knew he was worried. I could not tell him that I was curiously looking for this scent. He would think I was losing it. The fatigue became worse, and I no longer had the energy to locate that scent.

After I was admitted and transferred to my room, I thought I would be able to finally settle down. I was lying in bed on my back, falling asleep. Suddenly, I started seeing a beautiful light in the distance; it started off small, but it got brighter and closer. That scent I had searched for earlier was getting stronger, and it gave me so much peace. My respirations were more relaxed than they had been all day. I smiled because I could see two figures in the distance; they were somehow familiar and sparked my curiosity. I could see a white gown and a head full of long, black hair, but I could not clearly distinguish their facial features. My first impression of the forward figure was that it was a child, possibly a girl. Behind her, I saw an adult figure with a firmer jawline.

Even though the figures were close, I could not see their faces. I did not feel afraid by their presence—I felt comfort and was amazed by their beauty. The child figure extended her hand out to me, and I extended my right hand out to her. At that moment, I could feel myself lift off the bed. I felt as though I were floating easily above my bed. It was then that I realized I would leave this Earth. I did not want to leave my children there with just one parent. They were my responsibility too.

I pulled my hand back before our hands could touch and said, "I don't want to go. I wanted to stay to raise my children."

I did not want to leave them. If I had to go, though, I was prepared to do so.

I said, "If you let me stay, I will take care of your people."

I thought, *You cannot bargain with God*, but I could not bear leaving my children. Especially when I knew the pain of losing my own father when I was thirteen. I did not want them to feel the heartbreak I had felt. It was as though these spirits could read my thoughts. I don't know if I actually said the words, but gradually, the spirits left the room and the light went away.

The following morning, I heard a voice say, "You must have had some night."

I had not even realized there was another person in the room. A curtain was pulled between our beds, and she hadn't made a sound until then. Yes, it definitely was different.

She walked over to my bed and said, "Are you OK?"

I reassured her that I was fine. But I could tell by her concern she must have been present when I experienced the spirit's presence.

She said, "You were talking a lot last night. My name is Joyce. What is your name?"

I told her my name was Bernice.

"Nice to meet you, Bernice. Sounded like you were having some night," she replied.

She could tell I did not want to talk about it. I was still trying to process it myself. I needed to feel grounded; I realized my life could have ended, but I was grateful that God had allowed me to stay. I began to sob; tears of joy streamed down my face. I got up and went to the bathroom. I took one look at my face, and I realized my skin color still looked ashen. My eyes were streaked red, not just from crying but from the impact the asthma attack had had on my body. I continued to feel so weak. I wanted to shower, but I just didn't have the strength to do it. I got back into the bed quickly; even with the oxygen in use, I just couldn't muster up enough energy.

Just as I was returning to bed, the nurse entered the room and said, "You will be feeling better soon; you will be getting a lot of steroids."

Dr. Roberts stopped in to see me.

"Well, you gave us a lot of excitement last night," he said. "I am putting you on steroids three times a day. You are going to be here with us for several days to taper your dose. Let me listen to your lungs and heart. Still a lot of congestion going on in there, but we are going to take good care of you."

The nurse flushed my saline lock and slowly injected the steroids. I expected to have relief from the shortness of breath right away, which is what I had typically experienced. But I was so weak that I could barely get through the shower. I could forget about shampooing my hair; I just didn't have enough strength. I was forced to nap after the shower, which is something I never did. Just another reminder of how quickly things can change in a matter of minutes. After lunch, Arthur and my children came in for a visit. I was happy to see them. They both were smiling, but I could see that they were still a little anxious from the impact of seeing me in such a weakened state. We all hugged and kissed each other.

My husband said, "You have got to get well. Our son is having diarrhea, and he doesn't want to eat."

I knew I had to be strong for our children. My world revolved around them and their well-being. I had brought them into this world, and it was my responsibility to guide them.

After I had been in the hospital for a few days, my local family came to visit me—our friends and their families who also were not natives of the area. We formed our own support system by sharing progressive dinners, babysitting each other's children, and celebrating special events and holidays together. Their support and humor gave me strength and encouragement. The sisterhood that had developed over the years continues to have reverence with me.

The following day, I was finally able to return home. While I was at home, I had time to reflect on the gift of life I had been given. I decided I was not going to waste this gift, and I needed to be prepared to work for God. I had dedicated my life to God in a new way—and not just in prayer or by asking for help or for things in this world. Now it was my responsibility to wait, listen, and be obedient for what God needed me to do. I had the faith of a mustard seed and felt blessed to be given this opportunity. The change in mentation had begun.

My mother used to make mullein tea for me to treat respiratory illness. She would harvest the leaves and let them air dry in a mason jar. Maybe I should have never stopped drinking that tea.

——— BE NOT AFRAID BY JOHN TALBOT ———

"You shall cross the barren desert.
But shall not die of thirst.
You shall wander far in safety,
Though you do not know the way …

Be not afraid,
I go before you always,
Come follow Me …"

This song has always been my favorite, but now it had a new meaning. It was as if the words jumped off the page at me, which helped me to see these lyrics in a new way.

"And it is a good thing to receive wealth from God and the good health to enjoy it. To enjoy your work and accept your lot in life—this is indeed a gift from God." (Ecclesiastes 5:19, New Living Translation)

"Ask, and it shall be given you; seek, and ye shall find; knock, and it shall be opened unto you: For every one that asketh receiveth; and he that seeketh findeth; and to him that knocketh it shall be opened." (Matthew 7:7–8, King James Version)

I chose the first Bible verse because I enjoy being a part of the health-care team and helping to improve the quality of patients' lives. I was thankful for being able to heal from such an acute severe asthma attack, also referred to as status asthmatic-us. I chose the second verse because in the Bible, it says to ask for what we desire. I am glad that I thought to ask and that God allowed me to stay.

CHAPTER 7

Kappa Κκ: The Power of Nursing

Horsetail flower and nursing bind homeopathic benefits.

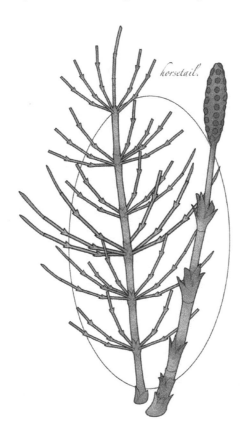

horsetail.

Horsetail flower is used to treat fluid-retention edema, kidney and bladder stones, urinary tract infections, incontinence (the inability to control urination), and general disturbances of the kidney and bladder.[7]

The Greek letter *kappa* means "something emerging from the core."

MRS. RUSSELL

When I returned to work, Mrs. Russell had been readmitted because of her chronic obstructive pulmonary disease. She had been a patient on our unit off and on for a couple years. Mrs. Russell was a sixty-two-year-old lady with a caramel skin tone and salt-and-pepper-colored hair. Her skin was bruised from the many needle sticks she had endured. She was a very robust woman of average stature. Her demeanor made her seem a little bit irritated, but deep down, she was tired, weak, and alone.

She was in the worst health state I had ever seen her. She was receiving IV vancomycin, steroids, and diuretics, but her shortness of breath was so exhausting for her that she always wanted to sleep and sit in the Geri chair, which is similar to a recliner, but it's on wheels and can lock. Sitting upright in that chair usually improved her lung expansion.

She was coughing up blood, and the pitting edema in her legs was not responding to the diuretics. Every day and night, Mrs. Russell spent all her time in the Geri chair, except when she needed to go to the bathroom or when we had her stand up to relieve the pressure off her buttocks and other body parts to prevent decubitus ulcers. After what I had just experienced, I could understand why she preferred sitting up. It created a straight line for airflow exchange of oxygen and carbon dioxide.

Mrs. Russell was a kind lady even when she felt bad, but this particular night, she seemed a little angry. The first thing she said was, "I have been waiting for you all day."

I thought, *I never work a day shift, so why were you waiting for me?* Then I thought maybe she'd had a bad day with the day-shift nurse and it had made her a little cranky. I washed her feet and applied moisturizers, because touch can heal and soothe both body and mind. Later that evening, the respiratory therapist came up to give her a nebulizer treatment, but Mrs. Russell did not seem to have much relief afterward. In fact, her use of accessory muscles—the rib cage; sternocleidomastoid muscle, which raises the rib cage; and neck muscles that move during times of abnormal or labored breathing—seemed to increase. I decided to check her vital signs to see if she was stable enough for an extra dose of Lasix, which usually helps to take the edge off the shortness of breath.

Her vital signs were: blood pressure 140/86, heart rate 92, respirations 28, and temperature 98.5. Her vitals were stable, so I called the hospitalist, who ordered Lasix 40 mg intravenous push for one dose. I also alerted April, the registered nurse I was working with, that I would need her to push the medication. April was such a good nurse, and she loved to teach. I pulled what we needed from the Pyxis medication dispensing machine and gathered the syringe and alcohol preps for her. We stood outside Mrs. Russell's room as she drew up the medication while standing by the medication cart. I informed Mrs. Russell of what medication April was going to give her and why. Mrs. Russell nodded to confirm that she understood what I was saying. April administered the medication and explained what she was doing.

As we were walking down the hallway, April said, "I can see why you called the hospitalist. She doesn't look good. This is a big change from yesterday."

I planned to ask her if it was OK to call her family to notify them of her change in condition and then see if she was willing to get in the bed. I would not want her sitting in that chair if we needed to transfer her to another unit." I knew she was a "do not resuscitate," but we still needed to keep her comfortable.

Twenty minutes later, the Lasix had begun to work. Her respirations were not as labored, and she seemed more comfortable. In the meantime, she agreed for me to call her family, but no one answered the telephone. I left a message for her sister to return my call as soon as possible. *Now is my window of opportunity to get her in the bed,* I thought.

"Mrs. Russell, I would like to get you into the bed and get you propped up with pillows so you can be more comfortable."

"OK," she said.

"Great. I am going to get everything I need, and I will be back shortly."

As I was leaving the room, I caught Barb in the hallway. "Please get some extra pillows to elevate Mrs. Russell's arms and legs. She has agreed to get in the bed."

"In the bed? She never gets in the bed," said Barbara.

"Yes, I know. That is why we must hurry so we don't miss our window of opportunity."

I called the security guards, Mike and Richard, to help with the transfer, because it had been a long day for her. Also, I wanted to make sure she was safe and that we had additional support personnel—just in case things took a turn for the worse. Mike and Richard came to the floor just as the phone rang at the nurse's station. It was Mrs. Russell's sister, returning my call. I informed her about the change in her respiratory status and that we had given her some Lasix to help ease her breathing.

Her sister said, "It's getting late. Do you think I should come in?"

"All I can tell you is that she asked me to call you and that she has been unsettled all evening."

"OK, I will come in," she said.

"Great. I will let security know so they will expect you. Just come through the emergency-room entrance."

The security guards and I headed to Mrs. Russell's room. As we entered, she laughed and smiled at me and stated, "You want to make sure I don't fall while getting into bed."

I smiled back at her and said, "I try to be prepared, and I want to make you as comfortable as possible."

We positioned her Geri chair right next to the bed. She only needed to stand briefly so that we could transfer her to the bed. Once she was sitting on it, I would lift her legs up into the bed while Barb managed her arms. The security guards stood on each side of her. Mrs. Russell had become frail and weakened over the years because of her disease process.

"Come on, fellows, let's do it," said Barbara.

We transferred her safely to the bed and started propping her up with pillows.

After we finished, she sighed and said, "That feels better," in a soft, gentle tone. Then she opened her eyes and said in a stern voice, "What is taking my sister so long?"

"I don't know," I said, "but I will go check."

I walked out, and I could see her sister at the end of the hallway. The security guards were boarding the elevator. I walked back into her room to announce that her sister was on the floor. But I noticed Mrs. Russell was very still and her chest was not rising. *Oh my God*, I thought. I used my stethoscope to assess her lungs and heart sounds, but neither were present. I adjusted her sheets and then started the long walk up the hallway, trying to get myself together.

I tried to think of what to say to her sister. Thoughts of my own sister flashed through my head. How would she have responded if this were me in the bed and she was coming to see me? As Mrs. Russell's sister approached me, I could see on her face the acknowledgment that something had happened.

She said, "She's already gone, isn't she?

I said, "She knew you had already endured enough pain, and she wanted to spare you from any more. You have been by her side comforting her so many times. This was the final gift she could give you, which was to spare you from enduring seeing her during those final moments."

I don't even know where those words came from, but I hoped they would help. Her sister sobbed for a few moments, and then she requested to see her. We prepared her body by removing the oxygen and any visible appliances so she would be in her natural state. Her sister was accompanied by her spouse, who embraced her.

After her sister left, we performed postmortem care and called security. The security officer said, "I think we were just in that room!"

"Yes, you are right; thank you for your help."

"She must have passed by the time we had gotten to the elevator."

"It was pretty close to that time," I replied.

Later that night, April said to me, "There must be something on you."

"What do you mean?"

"All of these patients keep dying when you're around," said April.

My eyes widened, and I said, "Oh, I had not really thought of it like that."

I began to think of the recent deaths on our floor. Not all the deaths had occurred when I was present, but more of them had than I'd realized. I began searching for an answer as to why this was happening; I loved my job, and I did not want anyone to think unfavorably of me.

After the morning shift report was over, I hurried off to see Father Daly at church. I knew he would be preparing for mass, and I wanted to catch him before it started.

If there was bad karma on me, he could bless me and relieve me from it. Reverend Daly had been a priest at Saint John for many years, and we had talked about many things over the years. I usually sat down and talked with him when it was time for confession because I knew my voice was familiar to him. When I arrived at church, I could see Father in the sacristy, preparing for mass.

I ran to his room and said, "Father, I need to ask you to bless me. My coworker said all these patients are dying when I am around."

Reverend Daly stopped what he was doing, looked me in the eyes, and said, "Did you do something wrong?"

I was surprised that he'd asked me that, but I knew it was his right to do so.

With a furrowed brow, I said, "No, Father."

He continued to adjust his vestments for mass. "So, let me just tell you that that you do not have that much power …"

His speech continued, but that was all I heard. I stood there, dazed, realizing the fact that nothing I had done had caused or changed the outcome of those patients' deaths.

Father stated, "OK, I'm going to bless you." He said a prayer over me and then stated, "I have to go to mass now, but if you want to talk more, come back."

I left the church feeling relieved but also a little confused. Why were these patients dying with me? I decided I needed to pay more attention. I started replaying in my mind what was happening before those patients died. Suddenly, it came to me. They had all said, "I was wondering if you were working tonight," or, "I have been waiting on you." I thought, *do people decide with or without God's intercession who will or will not be present when they take their last breath?*

I thought of my own experience. No one except the patient in the other bed had been present, but I had been unaware of her presence. There were no medical staff present when I felt the Lord coming for me. I was alone, but I did not want to leave this Earth.

I wondered how many of those people actually reached out to the Lord before they left this Earth and what that conversation might have been like. From a homeopathic perspective, there is still a lot of interest in horsetail as a diuretic, but current research shows that it reduces anxiety,[8] according to The National Center for Complementary and Integrative Health, U.S. National Institute of Health. I would have benefited from horsetail that day.

> "Because we know that the one who raised the Lord from the dead will also raise us with Jesus and present us with you to himself. All this is for your benefit, so that the grace that is reaching more and more people may cause thanksgiving to overflow to the glory of God. Therefore, we do not lose heart. Though outwardly we are wasting away, yet inwardly we are being renewed day by day." (2 Corinthians 4:14–16, New International Version)

> "Not only so, but we also glory in our suffering because we know that suffering produces perseverance; perseverance, character; and character, hope. And hope does not put us to shame, because God's love has been poured out into our hearts through the Holy Spirit, who has been given to us." (Romans 5:3–5, New International Version)

We know from the teaching of our Lord that we will all be raised from the dead to renew our commitment to our Lord and receive eternal life from Him. All the trials and tribulations we endure builds our strength and character—to give us hope for the future through the Holy Spirit, which has already been given to us. It is up to us to understand this.

CHAPTER 8

Omicron Oo: Peace

*Like motherwort manages heartbeats, Mrs. Brady
teaches us about matters of the heart.*

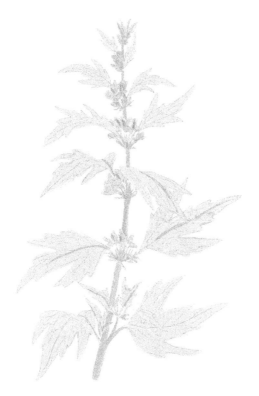

Motherwort manages heart failure and irregular heartbeat.[9]

The Greek letter *omicron* means "entity, intact entity," and "whole."

MRS. BRADY

Mrs. Brady transferred from another floor in the hospital to our unit. She had suffered a stroke and had regained very little cognitive function. The family was aware that her death was imminent. There was such peace with this patient and the family. She was a "do not resuscitate," so comfort measures were implemented such as oxygen, pain management, and nutrition as tolerated.

One or two family members kept vigil at her bedside at all times. They provided sips of water, cool cloths to her face, and soft strokes on her arms. It was obvious that this woman was very respected and loved by each one. They shared stories of how she had impacted their lives. You could see her smile from time to time, as though she were laughing or experiencing joy from hearing those stories being told.

During this time, the palliative care team at the hospital was creating a comfort cart for patients and family members. The cart contained glycerin mouth swabs, hard candy (usually for patients' guests), a variety of music, a radio/CD player, isolation gowns, gloves, various reading material, and quilts provided by the auxiliary staff.

Some of the standing orders for medications are morphine liquid, which is used to treat pain and shortness of breath; Ativan, which can be used to treat anxiety, nausea, or insomnia; and Levsin, an anticholinergic, or atropine, also used to treat wet respirations.

It is important to determine the patient's values, which helps provide insight to the staff on how to treat the patient holistically. Educating the family helps them gain insight about some of the symptoms that occur when a person is near the end of his or her life, such as: air hunger, which can be treated with morphine; terminal delirium, of which there are two types—hypoactive, which does not require treatment, and hyperactive, which is restless pulling at sheets or tubing, which can be treated with Haldol; the death rattle, which occurs when the saliva pools in the back of the soft palate (it is not uncomfortable for the patient but hard for the family to hear); and Cheyne-Stokes breathing, which is rapid, shallow breathing seen near the very end of life (it is difficult to medicate for this, but repositioning and other comfort measures should be continued).

Mrs. Brady did not speak but was able to use gestures to help the staff determine her needs. I could hear her family telling her, "It is OK to go." They said things like, "We appreciate everything you have done for us."

It is comforting to both the patient and the family to know that acceptance of impending death is shared. Mrs. Brady and her family were Catholic, and they actively practiced their beliefs. I asked them if they would like to have music played. I explained that music can be a sound of comfort, especially when playing comforting sounds such as religious songs or songs from the patient's favorite artists.

They decided on religious music. Mrs. Brady's granddaughter just happened to have a CD of *The Chaplet of Divine Mercy*, which is based on the Christological apparitions of Jesus reported by Saint Faustina Kowalska (1905–1938), known as "the Apostle of Mercy." She was a Polish religious sister of the Congregation of the Sisters of Our Lady of Mercy and canonized as a Catholic saint in 2000. According to Faustina's vision, the chaplet prayers for mercy are threefold: to obtain mercy, to trust in Christ's mercy, and to show mercy to others.

The Lord said to Blessed Faustina:

"You will recite this chaplet on the beads of the Rosary in the following manner:

First, you will say one Our Father, one Hail Mary, and then The Apostle's Creed.

Then, on the Our Father Beads you will say the following words:

'Eternal Father, I offer You the Body and Blood, Soul and Divinity of Your dearly beloved Son, Our Lord Jesus Christ, in atonement for our sins and those of the whole world"

On the Hail Mary Beads you will say the following words:

'For the sake of His sorrowful Passion,
have mercy on us and on the whole world"

In conclusion, three times, you will recite these words:

'Holy God, Holy Mighty One, Holy Immortal One,
have mercy on us and on the whole world.'

Our Lord said to Blessed Faustina: "Unceasingly recite this chaplet that I have taught you. Whoever will recite it will receive great mercy at the hour of death. Priests will recommend it to sinners as their last hope of salvation. Even the person who has grievously sinned, if he recites this chaplet even once, will receive grace from My infinite mercy. She wrote that Jesus said: ' ... When they say this Chaplet in the presence of the dying, I will stand between my Father and the dying not as the just judge but as the Merciful Savior.'"

As the CD was playing, you could see Mrs. Brady's shoulders start to relax, and her respirations became more at ease. I noticed that her family started to recite the prayer also. It is amazing how music can give someone peace.

Early that morning, Mrs. Brady surrendered to our Lord. Her family was at peace with her death and thanked the staff for their assistance with her care.

Mrs. Brady's death was peaceful. She had served her family and the Lord our God while she was on Earth. From the stories I heard, I am sure she is still doing God's work now. It is not necessary to give people food and fluids at the end of their life due to the potential for aspiration, which could lead to pneumonia. Sometimes that can be hard for family members to understand, but in reality, it can do more harm.

Motherwort manages an irregular heartbeat, which can cause a blood clot to form; a stroke caused the change in Mrs. Brady's mental status. Atrial fibrillation, or irregular heartbeat, is a factor of strokes among the elderly.

> "Jesus answered and said unto her, whosoever drinketh of this water shall thirst again. But whosoever drinketh of the water that I shall give him shall never thirst; But the water that I shall give him shall be in him a well of water springing up into everlasting life." (John 4:13–14, King James Version)

> "Let the peace of Christ rule in your hearts, since as members of one body you were called to peace. And be thankful." (Colossians 3:15 New International Version)

The first Bible verse is a metaphor about "well water" versus "living water," which is the Holy Spirit. Our desire for God should never end. As the second verse shows, being in a state of peace is our opportunity and possession when we believe and have a relationship with our Lord Jesus. I desire to have that peace with the Trinity. What about you?

CHAPTER 9

Psi Ψψ: Perception

Mr. Smith's perception could have been cleared by golden larch.

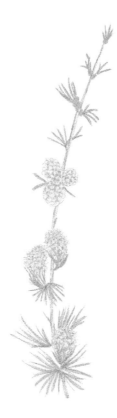

Pseudolarix amabilis is commonly known as golden larch, a member of the coniferous trees in the pine family. Golden larch is known to inhibit proliferation of cancer cells.[10]

The Greek letter *psi* means "incorporeal," or "without a body."

MR. SMITH

There was a gentleman named Mr. Smith who had a diagnosis of cancer of his pituitary gland. His primary physician consulted an oncologist, Dr. Steward, who informed the patient that his best option was chemotherapy with possible radiation. Each day that I worked while he was there, Mr. Smith would say to me, regardless of whether I was his nurse for that day or not, "I don't know what to do. I don't want to go through chemotherapy, but the doctor says it is the best option. Can you help me make a decision?"

"Oh, no, sir; I cannot do that. What I *can* do is to provide you with all the information about the chemotherapy and have the oncologist come back and speak with you."

"Oh, no; I don't like him. I don't trust him."

"We can have another oncologist give you a second opinion."

"I am sure it will just be the same news. Can I have my barber come in and give me a haircut?"

"Of course. We have a room set up for just that."

"Great, thank you. I am going to give him a call," said Mr. Smith.

"OK, I will check on you later. Just let me know if you need anything."

"OK," he replied. He waved goodbye to me as he dialed his barber's telephone number.

The next morning as I was making my rounds to check on every patient, I saw Mr. Smith in the hallway. He waved as he walked to the nurse's station. Upon my return up the hallway, I stopped and spoke to him.

"Good morning, Mr. Smith. How was your night?"

"It was all right. I just called my family. I asked them to come in later today," he said.

"OK, I will let you know when they arrive." I entered the room to check on Mr. Smith's roommate.

While I was talking to the patient in the first bed, Mr. Smith stood up and said, "I don't feel good."

"OK, Mr. Smith; lie down, please. I am going to check your vital signs."

The activities director, Sheila, was ambulating down the hallway, and I directed her to get the blood pressure machine while I pressed the room's call light to alert his nurse. Sheila returned with the blood pressure machine just as Mr. Smith clutched his chest and then took a deep breath. That was his last heartbeat and breath.

His nurse arrived at the bedside while I assisted the patient in the first bed out of the room. Mr. Smith was a "do not resuscitate." We were all taken aback at how quickly his condition had changed.

Just as we were placing a call to his family, his adult son arrived on the unit. He informed us that Mr. Smith had called the funeral home and made all his arrangements the previous day. We were all stunned by the news of Mr. Smith's awareness that he was dying.

An article titled, Herbal Active Ingredients: An Emerging Potential for the Prevention and Treatment for Papillary thyroid carcinoma, found that pseudolarix amabilis is known to suppress microtubule assembly to inhibit the proliferation, invasion, and migration of cancer cells.[11]

It is becoming more evident that homeopathic medication and traditional medication used as adjunct therapy should be considered as evidenced by continuing research.

I would be remiss if I did not tell you about the wonderful nine-year-old boy who read Bible verses to his paternal grandmother, who had raised the boy's father. I can only imagine how pleased she must have been to have experienced the love she had nurtured in her grandson and then flourished in her great-grandson. Love, faith, and respect encircled this family.

TO LIGHTEN YOUR HEART

In a hospital, staff members are challenged by people with a variety of personalities and unexpected reactions every day. I was taking care of an eighty-year-old female patient named Mrs. Wilson, who needed a Foley catheter inserted because it had been more than eight hours since she had voided (eliminated liquid waste, or urinated). After using the bladder scanner, I noted she had greater than 500cc of urine. Per the doctor's order and hospital protocol, I needed to insert the catheter to drain the bladder.

I went into the room to explain the procedure to her, and she acknowledged that she understood the rationale and procedure. I returned to the room with Garnett, a nursing assistant who would assist me, and with the required supplies. With each step, I explained everything to my patient, and her response was always, "OK." She allowed me to prep her peri area. Garnett was standing on the right side of the bed, and I was standing on the left. Just as I was starting to insert the Foley, her left leg swung up on my shoulder. *I need to hurry up,* I thought.

Garnett's eyes widened, but she remained at Mrs. Wilson's right side. "I am almost done, Mrs. Wilson. I just need to inflate the balloon." Mrs. Wilson extended her hand out to Garnett, and somehow she flung her right leg up. Now both of her legs were on my shoulders. Garnett just stood there, looking straight ahead and holding Mrs. Wilson's hand.

I continued to reassure her, while also trying hard to stand up straight to help her legs fall off my shoulders. But she was squeezing so tightly with her legs that she started to draw me down closer to the bed. One of the day-shift nurses came in to see what was taking so long because she was ready for report. As she entered the room, she started to snicker.

"Oh my, would you like some help?"

"Yes, as you can see. I have lost my helper."

Garnett looked at me and started laughing as she shook her head. The day-shift nurse was able to get her legs off my shoulders, and then I stabilized the Foley catheter tubing to Mrs. Wilson's leg.

When I came out of the room, Chantel, another nursing assistant, started talking in our departmental director's tone of voice, who she loved to imitate all the time.

"Bernice, can you tell me what went wrong with Foley catheter insertion?"

Chantel had mastered her body gestures as well. We all died laughing.

▪ ONE OF MANY HUMOROUS COWORKERS ▪

Mr. Smithy, a housekeeper, was a very kind soul who enjoyed making people laugh. He would get so tickled about what he was thinking that he could barely tell the joke. He was a devout Christian who would challenge anyone to understand the purpose of faith. One of his favorite jokes was:

"Knock, knock."

"Who's there?"

"Luke."

"Luke who?"

"Luke through the peephole and find out!"

His jokes were always corny but distracted us—in a good way—from the events of the day. We always looked forward to seeing him. He was a dependable worker.

> "Fear not, for I am with you; be not dismayed, for I am your God; I will strengthen you, I will help you, I will uphold you with my righteous right hand." (Isaiah 41:10, New King James Version)

> "For God so loved the world, that He gave His only begotten Son, that whoever believes in Him shall not perish, but have eternal life." (John 3:16, New International Version)

I am so grateful for the teaching of God. He has created all of us. He desires for us to call on him at all times in our lives. Are you asking for your gifts that God has for each of us?

CHAPTER 10

Pi Ππ: Acknowledgment

*Mrs. Rogers commands attention just as licorice
commands acknowledgment.*

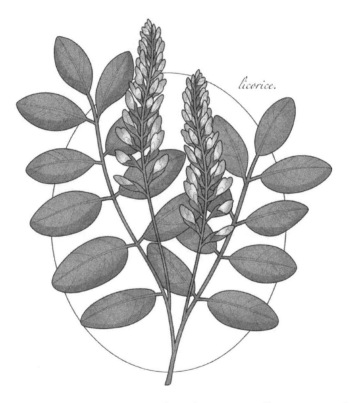

licorice.

Licorice root is a potent antioxidant that is anti-inflammatory and has antimicrobial effects. It may ease upper respiratory infections, treat ulcers, and aid in digestion.[12]

The Greek letter *pi* means "unified; under the same roof."

MRS. ROGERS

Mrs. Rogers was a seventy-five-year-old female with end-stage renal disease. She had a wonderfully supportive daughter named Jennifer, who was her mother's right hand. When Mrs. Rogers arrived at the unit, her daughter pulled out a list of her medications and recent laboratory values.

Mrs. Rogers said, "Please don't mind her. She thinks she is my personal nurse."

Jennifer said, "Oh, Mom, you know I am just doing what is best for you."

Mrs. Rogers said, "She thinks she can save me, but the truth is, when it is time, it is time, and I am getting tired."

"Mom, stop talking like that," said Jennifer.

Mrs. Rogers looked at her daughter and realized her words were upsetting her.

She changed the subject and said, "What's on the menu for today? I would really love to have a cup of coffee. Jennifer, I know you need to take Charles for his appointment. Go home and get some rest; I will see you tomorrow."

Garnett and I helped Mrs. Rogers settle in for the evening. She was suffering from sepsis related to kidney disease, and she had a nephrostomy tube on her left back to drain her urine. A nephrostomy tube is inserted into your kidney posteriorly with a valve that has three openings. One of the openings is attached to the tubes, another is attached to a drainage bag, and the last one is attached to an irrigation port.

The next evening as Garnett and I entered Mrs. Rogers's room, she was gazing at the wall. She did not acknowledge our presence at first, but then she turned to me and said, "God said that you are going to be with me when I die. No one else, just you. He loves you."

Garnett turned to me and said, "What's happening?"

"I don't know; just go with it. Let her talk."

Some of her words were unclear to me; she turned her head and nodded as if someone was speaking to her. I asked Garnett to get the blood pressure cuff so we could check her vital signs. I could tell that whatever was going on, it was giving her comfort and peace. Her vital signs were stable, so Garnett and I left the room to allow her time to finish this journey she was clearly experiencing. I realized she was having a conversation with God, and I wanted her to do so comfortably.

As the days went by, Mrs. Rogers's nephrostomy tube started to decrease the amount of urine it was draining. I contacted the doctor. His order increased the amount of saline used to flush her tube. Despite our efforts, her kidney output function continued to decline. As her kidney function decreased, so did her interactions with her family and staff. Her daughter would come to visit and sit without her mother acknowledging her presence at times. But then other days, she would interact with her and talk about pleasant experiences they had shared together in the past. A few days later when I returned to work, I was making my rounds, checking on everyone.

When Mrs. Rogers saw me, she said, "I was wondering if you were coming back to work. I haven't seen you in a few days."

Oh, that was my cue. *I need to hurry up and finish what I need to do, because I have a feeling she is going to need me.* Our shift started at seven p.m., and at around 8:30, I could see that her respirations and mentation continued to decrease gradually. I asked her if I could call her daughter, and she said yes. I moved quickly to get her daughter on the phone, and she agreed to come in. I went back to her room and sat in the chair next to her and held her hand.

My coworker Kia walked by the room. "Oh, I know what you are doing. I couldn't do that, but do you need anything?" she said.

"Just make sure everyone is OK. Garnett knows where I am, but she might need some help."

"OK, I will check on her," said Kia.

Mrs. Rogers never reopened her eyes. She would sigh deeply when I repositioned her, which made me question whether I was annoying her or interrupting something. But she always resumed her comfortable position. She rested like an infant who was being turned while sleeping peacefully—that's what it reminded me of. I was beginning to watch the clock more closely now. It had been a little while since I had called her daughter, and she had not arrived yet. I was beginning to feel a little nervous because I was afraid she was not going to make it.

Then I remembered the conversation Mrs. Rogers and I had had on the first day we'd met. I took a deep breath and acknowledged that I was to be here until the end. I sat by her side and held her hand until her respirations ceased and her heartbeat stopped. I turned off the support systems and started down the hallway. I looked up and saw her daughter, Jennifer, walking quickly toward me.

She said tearfully, "She couldn't wait for me."

I could see the pain on her face. "I don't think she wanted you to endure that pain. You had given so much of yourself that she wanted your last memory of her to be good."

Jennifer said, "I could have taken it. She cheated me of this."

Wow, I was not expecting that response. I was emotionally and physically drained, so it took me a moment to come back with a response. I explained, "It is not easy to watch your loved one gradually leave this Earth, and she wanted to spare you from that agony."

She took one look at me and then hugged me and thanked me for being at her mother's side and apologized for her words. I acknowledged her pain, but I never mentioned that her mother had told me that only I would be by her side at the end. I did not want to hurt her.

For reasons unknown to us, God always has a plan. I have learned to just go with it. Because if we try to intercede, we usually just make a mess of things. Jennifer was able to gather her composure and visit with her mother for a few minutes. But before she left, she gave me a copy of the preferred funeral home and other important details for her postmortem care. Mrs. Rogers did not want to be an organ donor. However, in the state of Maryland, we are required to contact the Living Legacy Foundation. Her body was denied based on her last lab values, recent diagnosis, and age.

Licorice is used to treat inflammation. Inflammation is a biological response of the body's tissues to pathogens, damaged cells, or irritants, which involves a protective response from the body that stimulates immune cells to clear out the cells that are damaged and start the repair process. The kidneys are our filtering organs.

During one Sunday sermon during mass, we heard that God says in the Bible, "I will put my spirit in you for those who believe." Even mortal death does not bring death to our soul. God's love is so great that it is far beyond death itself. Do you believe that God is the resurrection and the light? Death is not the end for those who believe. God has power over death itself. The reality of physical death has no power, if only the spirit of God dwells in you. We go to God for the gift of mercy. All we need to do is allow God into our lives. God waits for us to invite him into our lives.

> "My sheep hear my voice, and I know them, and they follow me: And I give unto them eternal life; and they shall never perish, neither shall any man pluck them out of my hand." (John 10:27–28, King James Version)

> "For he that speaketh in an unknown tongue speaketh not unto men, but unto God: for no man understandeth him; howbeit in the spirit he speaketh mysteries." (1 Corinthians 14:2, New King James Version)

To me, the first Bible verse means that God enables those who seek and follow his teaching with the ability to hear him. The second Bible verse reflects on tongues, of how God is able to communicate between individuals and himself.

I began to have a greater understanding of the importance of being content with when my own end of life would come. I can only imagine how much comfort Mrs. Rogers must have felt, knowing how her life would end.

CHAPTER 11

Tau Tτ: Be true to Thy Own Spirit

Mrs. Wilson, like most of us, would benefit from St. John's wort.

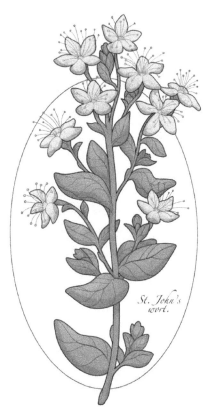

St. John's wort.

St. John's wort is used to treat depression.[13]

The Greek letter *tau* means "tension-force" or "stretch/extend."

MRS. WILSON

Mrs. Wilson was going to arrive at our unit for end-of-life care. She was an oncology patient whose health was complicated with multiple comorbidities. When she arrived, her eyes were wide, blinking, and roaming around the room. She was nonverbal, and her demeanor was anxious, rigid, and tense, as though she was afraid. I thought this would change once she became accustomed to our voices and the surroundings. But her demeanor never changed; it actually became more intense. Her respirations were not labored, her heart rate was in the nineties, and her blood pressure was stable.

The doctor ordered the regular end-of-life care medications for comfort, related to her status of "do not resuscitate" and referral for hospice. She was given Ativan per the doctor's order. Her family—her brother, sister, and spouse—remained at her side. The family was quiet and did not want to engage with the staff.

When we attempted to ask questions or explain procedures before implementing them, the response was, "Just do what you have to do." This was unusual behavior, because most of our clients want to know what is going on and how we plan to care for their loved one. There was a tenseness in the air. I tried to figure out what was causing this strained environment.

Later, her brother revealed that they had just lost their mother and had not dealt with the loss. I spoke about the support systems available, but it seemed as though they did not want any support at that time. They did not speak to one another; they just sat there as though they were numb. The loss of multiple family members can be traumatic. Each person deals with the end of life differently. As nurses, we are taught to nurture our clients and their families; this type of interaction was foreign to me.

I continued to provide care for Mrs. Wilson, turning and repositioning her, swabbing her mouth as needed. While we were in the room, there was an eerie feeling that made me uncomfortable. I had no fear of being around someone who was dying. But it felt as though there was a negative presence there. Her family decided to leave. After they left, Mrs. Wilson began to gaze even more at the ceiling, and her facial expression was one of fear.

I asked April to give her some Ativan. As we were approaching the room, the bed started to shake. There was no one in the room. The shaking had to come from Mrs. Wilson. We stood there dumbfounded; neither one of us had even seen anything like that in our lives. When the bed stopped shaking, she was no longer on this Earth. Oh my—that was one of the scariest things I have witnessed in my career. When it was time to perform postmortem care, we usually closed the door completely for privacy. However, we did not feel comfortable doing that; luckily for us, the timeframe of her death was at night, which allowed for a lot less foot traffic on our unit and also allowed us to perform the care alone with the door slightly ajar.

I felt as though this person might not have known or had a relationship with God. I wondered if in her last moments, she was seeing things she had never believed in or had ever thought about.

> "For I am convinced that neither death, nor life, nor angels, nor principalities, nor things present, nor things to come, nor powers, nor height, nor depth, nor any other created things, will be able to separate us from the love of God, which is in Christ Jesus our Lord." (Romans 8:38–39, New International Version)

> "Yea, though I walk through the valley of the shadow of death, I will fear no evil; for thou art with me; thy rod and thy staff they comfort me."(Psalms 23:4, King James Version)

The first Bible verse has been described as the first death and as embracing our body, soul, and spirit. Psalms 23:2 acknowledges that when we are afraid, God reminds us that he is always protecting and guiding us. God is always offering us a place of peace and rest.

CHAPTER 12

Omega Ωω: Mother

A mother's love leads the head of our hearts.

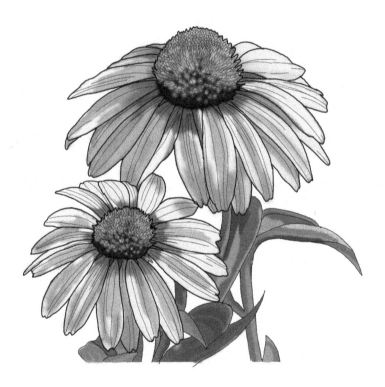

Echinacea flower reduces inflammation, improves immunity, and lowers blood sugar levels.[14]

The Greek letter *omega* means "bring forth" and "the end."

MOTHER

On Sunday, May 16, my mom called. I thought she was calling to have our usual chat. But to my surprise, she said, "I am scheduled to have a lung biopsy in less than two weeks."

I did not hear what my family was talking about in the background. I could only deal with what my mother was saying to me. Then I started to hear my husband say something to me, but I could not respond to him. I put my hand up and pointed to the phone to indicate that I needed to listen.

"Mom, I will be there for your test."

"I am sorry for the late notice," said Mom.

"Try not to worry about that. You just found out this week. I am just glad you let me know. I want to be there for you."

In my head, I was thinking, *Oh no*. My mother had received a diagnosis of colon cancer and had a portion of her colon surgically removed many years ago. I briefly thought about the potential for the cancer to reoccur again. The question was, was that time now?

After I finished speaking with my mother, Arthur told the kids, "Watch your mother. She is not thinking clearly. She has a lot on her mind." I thought I was OK, but I was wrong. I had cut my finger with the butcher knife, and I did not even realize it until I saw the blood.

Arthur walked over, took me by the hand, and said, "Let's go upstairs. You need a Band-Aid and some peroxide."

I knew I needed stitches, but I did not have time for that. I needed to plan my trip to Kentucky and also notify my job that I would need time off.

My mother had had a severe reaction to anesthesia and pain medication before, which caused her to require an emergency trach placement after esophageal swelling. I felt as though I needed to be there this time, just in case.

I realized that this was the start of a journey I did not want to take. But I knew I could not stop it either. I had been so supportive to my patients over the years, and now it was my turn to be there for my mother. My son and daughter decided they would help me drive to Kentucky. We packed our bags and planned to leave that Saturday.

I received a call from my brother Tommy. He said, "Mom has been diagnosed with lung cancer. You know if she has it there, then she probably has it everywhere."

My brother Bobby received a diagnosis of prostate cancer on May 20—the same day my mother received her diagnosis. I went to work that night because I needed to stay busy to occupy my mind. After that night, I was off for a few days, so during that time, I prayed and asked God for guidance.

On Thursday, Bobby called and said, "Mom is having a lot more pain and coughing up blood."

On Friday morning, Tommy called and said, "I think you better come home."

I shared the information from the conversations I'd had with my brother with my children and Arthur. We decided to leave the next day. Bobby was already at Mom's house when we arrived.

He greeted us at the door. "I am glad you made it. You really need to be here."

Mom had stopped coughing up the blood and was settling down. I needed to calm myself, so Sunday morning, my family and I headed off to church while Bobby stayed with Mom. Once at Saint Dominic Catholic Church, they were singing my favorite song, "Be Not Afraid." My family had attended mass at this church for many years, since before I was born. The church was only a ten-minute drive, if that, from my mother's home. They announced my mother's name along with other parishioners who were ill and needed prayers.

Later that afternoon, we went to visit my nephew and pay our respects to him and his wife's family. His wife had always brought out the best in him. While we were visiting my nephew, my Aunt Betty and her grandson arrived. Just before dinner, Mom started to have pains in her chest, and she asked us to pray for her. I used blessed oil from Jerusalem to make the sign of the cross on Mom, and we began with our prayers, each one praying to God what was on our hearts.

Blessed oil, a sacramental like holy water, helps the faithful to grow in their spiritual life and increases their devotion to the Catholic faith. It can be used to bless oneself or another person, as a healing balm, and as protection against evil. Blessed oil is not the same as "holy oils."

The next day, I could hear my mother in the shower at four a.m. I entered her room to help her finish up. She was in good spirits and ready for her procedure. She went back to bed to rest until seven. Aunt Betty, Tommy, Bobby, Art, Junior, Jessica, and I left the house by eight a.m.

After the biopsy, the nurse called us to come to her recovery area to be at my mother's bedside. I could tell she was struggling a little to breathe; her entire chest was moving. I thought, *Give her a moment.*

The doctor came to her bedside and stated, "I was not able to do the biopsy." He paused and put his head down. "It was just too vascular, and each time I tried to get a specimen, the site would bleed. So I had to stop."

"Is that what you would have done with your own mother?" asked my brother.

I took my elbow and poked him side to get him to calm down. He just looked at me and said, "No."

"I think she is having difficulty breathing, which I am more concerned about at this time. Can someone check her pulse oximetry?" I said.

I was more concerned about her oxygen saturation than the biopsy at this point. In my mind, he had just told us that it was inoperable. My goal now was to do whatever it took to keep her comfortable. That comfort began with her respirations being unlabored. I asked the doctor if he thought the bleeding could be continuing or if he was able to stop it. Knowing that she had stopped taking her blood thinner for the procedure, I was concerned that she might not have stopped the medication in time. Her O_2 saturation was 88 percent on room air. They applied oxygen via the nasal cannula at two liters. The nurse in me showed up.

I said, "Don't you think you should do a chest x-ray and check her electrolytes because she has a tendency to lose potassium?"

"I have no idea how long the fluids have been infusing and at what rate." The doctor took one look at me as if to say that I was out of line. I knew I had overstepped my boundaries, but the patient was my mother—not a stranger.

Now her oxygen saturation was 84 percent.

I looked at the nurse and said, "She needs a venti-mask."

Just then, the anesthesiologist came in and ordered Lasix 20 mg IV and a chest x-ray. The chest x-ray showed pulmonary edema. Pulmonary edema, when sudden, can lead to respiratory failure or cardiac arrest due to hypoxia. But through it all, Mom remained calm; the wheezing sound coming from her lungs was audible without a stethoscope. After the Lasix started working, her oxygen saturations started to increase to 91 percent and finally to 94 percent at best on four liters via a regular face mask. Before that, her oxygen saturation was 98 percent on room air.

The original plan was for her to be discharged after the procedure, but given the change in her respiratory status, the doctor decided to admit her to ICU room seven. My family and I left the hospital. I was disappointed, sad, and frustrated, not to mention ready to cry. My mother was eighty-two years old, and I knew the potential for her condition to change quickly was always a possibility.

When we arrived at my mother's home, my brother said, "You know Mom has had cancerous cells in the past."

I did not want to talk about it. I just sat there and listened to him go on and on. I knew he had to release everything he had been thinking about or else neither one of us would get any rest. I was both physically and emotionally fatigued.

Later that evening, we went back to the hospital, and Mom's breathing was less laborious. She acknowledged that she wasn't ready to leave yet. She laughed about how bad the chicken was and said that she could only eat a few potatoes. Mom's oxygen saturations were maintained at 94 percent on four liters.

Later that night, Aunt Betty, Tommy, Bobby, and I sat down and had a conversation about planning for Mother's care. None of us wanted Mom to go to a nursing home, so we planned to provide her care at home. We decided to split day, night, and the weekends. I knew this was not going to last for long. Somehow, life worked it out that I was able to come home for a week every three weeks to give them a break.

The following morning before we went to pick up Mom from the hospital, our goal was to get her set up with all the things she would need, so that my brothers could just focus on being with her. I washed clothes and organized her clothing for comfort. I organized her kitchen cabinets and grocery items. Once Mom arrived home, I could see some anxiety on her face. She knew I was planning on leaving in a few days. My heart was torn; I knew my children had to get back to school, but I really felt like I needed to stay.

That night, Mom started having chest pain. I gave her the prescribed OxyContin for pain; then I prayed for relief of her pain. My mother prayed every day, all throughout the day. When I was growing up, I went to church twice a week when school was in session. I attended a Catholic school from first to eighth grade, and then on Sunday, we went to mass. If there were any holy days of obligation, we were present for the ceremony—not to mention, we prayed the rosary as a family during the week. My mother was a member of the Franciscan Order of Divine Compassion's Third Order, also known as the Brothers and Sisters of Penance.

By the time we had finished praying, she started to feel better. The next day, the family and Mom decided it was time to call hospice for a consultation. But first we had to contact Dr. Shula, Mom's primary-care physician. When I spoke to him on the phone, he seemed just as anxious as I was. He had been my mother's doctor for over twenty years. He spoke to my mother to tell her that if the pain became worse during the night, we should just take her to the hospital.

Dr. Shula gave orders for oxygen and pain management for home use. The hospice nurse arrived and brought oxycodone for her pain. Mom was able to eat what she had requested for dinner: blackened fish, baked sweet potatoes, and broccoli. Her grandsons and cousin came by to visit, which brought a smile to her face. Mom loved her family and friends. Later that night, I lit a blessed candle, usually lit for prayer intentions, hoping for peace for all of us.

I felt relief to have the hospice nurse to share information with and she would be able to alert me of significant changes in Mom. I had been able to be at the bedside to help so many people before they departed this earth. I asked God to let me be there with my own mother. I lived twelve hours away by car, so I knew that presented a challenge, but I had the faith of a mustard seed.

On July 27, I returned to Kentucky to be with Mom. I worked on cleaning her house while she slept. Mom was eating well, but she was weaker. She ambulated to the bathroom alone but had to stop and sit in a chair before returning to her bed. I could tell she was having more pain; she had also taken three pain pills that day, which was a lot for her. Mom would pray and offer her pain up to God.

To complicate matters, hospice withdrew from providing care due to miscommunication. I had to have Mom reinstated. While waiting for their call, I received a call from my girlfriend Theresa back home. She had just been diagnosed with breast cancer, and one lymph node had also come back positive for cancer cells. Oh, my goodness—no, this couldn't happen to my friend. She had so much vitality. She had been so helpful to so many people, but now it was time for her to focus on herself. Theresa is the type of person who just randomly pays for someone's groceries while standing in line behind them. I took a walk after that conversation and prayed. *Lord, I know my mom is weak, but not my friend too, please.*

When I returned, Mom said, "I just need more time."

Oh no, Mom is beginning to feel different, I thought. I sat down beside her and just hugged her and tried to hide my tears. This was hard because I knew she was aware of how much she was changing. I did not want her to focus on her end of life, but we both knew and realized that the cancer was getting worse. I tried to change our thoughts and asked Mom what she would like for dinner. She said baked fish, green beans, and sliced tomatoes. Thank goodness—whatever I fixed, she seemed to enjoy it. Some cancer patients develop a metallic taste or lose the desire to eat all together.

Mom said, "I feel like you say prayers for me all the time."

"I try to, Mom."

I actually had been praying for my mother, but even more so during that time. I thought it was amazing that she could sense my prayers. Mom's acknowledgment of my prayers was just a confirmation of her relationship with God. My mom was so good to so many people. She worked for Community Action passing out food, clothing, and subsidized aid. She worked at the local library reading stories to the children and checking out the library books—not to mention all the loving things she did for her family.

Mom's insurance provided a nursing assistant named Felecia, who came during the day for a few hours.

Felecia said, "The seasons will be changing soon. We need to switch your clothes from summer to fall."

Felecia would assist Mom with her ADLs, short for activites of daily living, throughout the week, plus she was a friend of the family. It provided me comfort knowing that she was cared for and that Felecia would not hesitate to call me if she had any concerns.

We cleaned out the drawers and separated the clothing. Mom was the overseer, of course. It was reassuring to have her directing us as to how and where she wanted her belongings. She was accustomed to announcing exactly where each item of clothing was located without being present in the room.

One day, I took my cousin Tina with me for Mom's follow-up appointment with her oncologist. Mom had a lung scan while I was away. She said she did not want to go for the follow-up appointment because she was feeling weak. When we arrived at the office, the nurse took us to a regular exam room. When the doctor entered the room, I introduced my cousin.

He acknowledged her presence and then said, "The cancer has spread since the procedure, and this is an aggressive cancer, stage four. There is no treatment for this. We will do whatever we can to keep her comfortable."

My heart dropped. I waited until I got into the car, and I sobbed.

I thanked Tina for going with me; that would have been hard to hear alone. When I arrived home, I told Mom what the doctor had said.

She said, "I don't want you to cry over me, because you have had me for a very long time. And if you cry, it will change the way your children handle it. You have to be strong for your family. Because if there is any way I can come back to you and help you, I will."

I could tell Mom was trying to prepare my mindset because she could feel the changes within herself. My mom was dear to me. I loved my own family as well, but the love of a mother is special and unconditional. I was fortunate to have had a mother who supported me in everything I ever wanted to do. I remember when I was getting married, she told me to write down everything I wanted on my wedding day and not to hold anything back.

Mother provided meals for the visiting priest at Saint Dominic's Parish. Father Hayden, Mother, and the church secretary had developed a friendship. One evening, Mother was reading my letter at work in the presence of Father Hayden, who said, "Who does she think she is?"

My mom smiled, laughed, and said, "I told him she knows exactly who she is. She is Robert and Juanita Wright's daughter."

Father Hayden is a kind spirit who ended up presiding over my wedding ceremony. Priests are held in high regard, and Mother respected Father Hayden, but she supported her children. I don't even remember what it was I wanted to do. I do remember how sought-after Father Hayden was. When he performed wedding ceremonies, no one ever separated or divorced.

Mom woke up early, around 4:30 in the morning. I awoke to find her in the bathroom sitting on the toilet. She had an incontinent episode, which my mother never had. She agreed to take a shower, so I placed the shower chair and set up the bathroom. Mom was able to transfer to the tub, but I could tell that she did not feel well. I went to the oxygen concentrator and added some extension tubing so she could relax while showering since it would reduce her fatigue.

During the night, I decided I needed to sleep in her room. I brought the bedside commode to her room to decrease the number of steps she had to take to the bathroom.

Mom said, "If there is anything here you want, take it back with you. I know what everyone else wants. I have already given them (my siblings) some things, and the rest is written down in that book."

Mom always kept holy water on her bedside table. I was going to refill it because it was almost empty, but now it was full to the top. No one was in the house with us that I was aware of. How did that bottle get full again? I blessed Mom and myself, making the sign of the cross with the holy water for peace. I prayed that God would help us make the right choices.

Mom said, "I know all of you will miss me, but Tommy and you will have the hardest time. You have to be strong."

Aunt Betty called to check on her sister. Mom said frankly, "I have cancer and they can't cure it. I am worried about Tommy. He left a while ago, and he hasn't slept much." I could hear the directness and fear in her voice.

The fear was a side of my mother I don't think I had ever seen. I told Mom I would check on Tommy while I was out at the grocery store. I started playing some family videos after her telephone conversation to preoccupy her mind. My sister Laura and I had planned for our sister Elizabeth to come and visit with Mom. Elizabeth had moved to another town to be close to her children after she retired.

It had been a while since they had seen each other. Elizabeth and Mom had worked together for several years doing community service work. They shared similar hobby interests and spent a lot of time together at church and family functions. Elizabeth was beginning to have a decrease in appetite, and so was Mom. Many years of various health issues had begun to take a toll on Elizabeth's body. While they were en route, I prepared a Southern meal of fresh fried chicken, mashed potatoes, gravy, fresh green beans, garden sliced tomatoes, iced tea, and peach cobbler for dessert.

The two of them sat in that kitchen and talked, laughed, and ate like we had not seen either one of them do in months. When they decided it was time for rest, Elizabeth hugged my mother as if she knew it might be the last time their paths would cross on this Earth. It gave Pearl and I so much joy to see the two of them together, but also a little heartbreak because of what was to come.

My parents had fourteen children between the two of them. My father had ten by his first wife, who died early in life. My mother had two children by her first husband. When my parents married, they had two more children. So there are lots of cousins, nieces, and nephews. We were blessed with a large family, and our family was taught to help each other. I had made arrangements for my great-niece Tanita to spend nights with Mom because I could see this was taking a toll on my brothers. Even though I was coming home every three weeks to give them all a break and staying for at least a week, this was beginning to take a toll on us all. I was still working full time while trying to manage her care, her household needs, and my own household as well.

Mom called me one evening while Tanita was there. "Why are you making this child stay here with me?" she asked.

"You need company, and I want to make sure you are not alone."

"I appreciate what you are trying to do, but you don't have to worry about me. I will be fine. She needs to be at home resting with her own children," said Mom.

"Mom, it gives me comfort knowing someone is there with you."

"So, you are going to keep on having her come by?"

"Yes, Mom. When I am at home, she will not have to be there."

"So when are you coming home?"

"Soon, I will call you with the dates tomorrow, OK?"

"All right; good night."

"I love you, Mom. Good night."

On September 27, I received a telephone call from the hospice nurse, Ruby.

She said, "You need to come home. Your mother has changed. She has three-plus edema and looks dusky."

I was with my husband at a fundraiser golf tournament when I received the call. I asked the Lord to please let me make it home to be at my mother's side when she left this Earth. I thanked the Lord for the gift of being present with patients when they were passing. I found my husband and told him about the phone call. During the drive home, I felt like a lump was in my throat. Once I arrived at home, I started looking for flights. I was able to get an afternoon flight for the next day. I had to work that night, so I asked Jessica to drive me to the airport.

It started raining hard late that night; by morning, it was still raining. I went to the basement to check the floor because we'd had water leak under the door in the past, especially with excessive amounts of rain. It had been raining off and on for several days that week, so the ground was saturated. Of course, there was a small amount of water on the floor. There was no way I could rest after seeing the water on the floor. I just started using the shop vac to suck up the water; then I disinfected the floor and shoe molding. Thank goodness Jessica was able to drive me to the airport.

After showering, I rested for thirty minutes before it was time to leave for the airport. My flight was delayed due to the weather. Once I landed in Kentucky, I drove to Mom's house. When I arrived, Mom was lying in the hospital bed in her room, and she was short of breath. I could hear her wheezing. My brothers were at her bedside. We all hugged one another. Mom was awake most of the night, attempting to pull her oxygen off. I slept for only two and half hours at most. I tried singing church songs with her, and then I started singing another song.

Mom said, "It's OK if you just want to read the Bible." I died laughing because I knew that was her way of saying, "You can't sing." The look she gave me was a look of surprise that such an out-of-tune tone was coming out of me, especially because my mother sang in the church choir for many years. I guess she was wondering how it was possible that I was unable to carry a tune. Later that afternoon, Mom was sitting up in the bed looking out the window, smiling. She moved to the bottom of the bed and pulled the curtains back.

I asked her, "What do you see that is making you so happy?"

Mom said, "I see my mom and dad coming to get me."

I had to fight back the tears because she had already told me that she needed me to be strong. I sat down next to her and stroked her hair and looked out that window with her. I tried to hide the tears streaking down my face because I realized my mom was slipping away from us.

The next day, I made a brief trip to the store to restock supplies for my mother. While I was out, I received a call from the hospice nurse, who wanted to insert an indwelling catheter into Mom because she was retaining urine. I agreed. Shortly after her call, I received a second call from the nurse who stated, "I can't get the catheter in."

I thought, *Wow, I am going to put the indwelling catheter in.* I knew I'd have to, because if my mother was complaining about it, it must have really been irritating her. I told the nurse I was only ten minutes away from the house and that if she would stay, I would be there to insert the catheter. I brought the items into the house. I washed my hands, donned the sterile gloves, and started the procedure. Sometimes in women, the bladder shifts, so you have to take a nontraditional approach to insert the catheter. Dark amber urine was in the tubing. I knew then that Mom was dehydrated and probably had a urinary tract infection.

The nurse said, "She told me she is having a hard time pivoting to use the bedside commode. I think she is weaker than she is letting on."

It was a lot for Mom to have me insert the indwelling catheter, but I could see the relief on her face as her bladder emptied. Renee, our mother's neighbor who is a nurse and routinely checked in with Mom, called and wanted to come over to help Mom get settled for the night.

"Hello, Mrs. Juanita."

Mom had an endearing smile as soon as she heard Renee's voice. Renee would comb and French braid my mother's hair. I decided to turn the television on, just in case Mom wanted to share something with Renee privately. Plus, Mom normally had the TV on.

Mom said, "Play something I want to watch."

I began to notice some intermittent frustration from Mom. I thought her pain must be getting worse. Some Christians believe you should offer your pain and or suffering up to the Lord for what he has endured for us.

Later, she told me, "I saw Julia and my aunt Mary." They are both deceased. "I am sorry I have been angry. Just …"

Oh no, my mother must be in pain, I thought. I gave Mom her prescribed pain medication so she could get some relief and finished helping her get ready for bed.

"Mom, you have to tell us when you are having pain, so we can give you something for it.

She took a deep breath and continued adjusting herself in the bed. I knew that meant "I will let you know when I want you to know." Aunt Betty decided it was time to come see her sister while she could engage in conversation.

The next morning, I told Mom, "Your sister is coming to see you today."

Later in the day, Aunt Betty called to say she was having a difficult time finding someone to stay with her husband. His health was declining also, and she did not want to leave him alone. She had finally found someone and was on her way. After I got off the phone, I told Mom she was on her way.

Mom said, "I've been hearing that all day!"

Bobby and I looked at each other and walked hurriedly out of the room. This was a side of Mom we normally did not see. We thought it was best to give her some time alone. We did not want to frustrate her. Or was she waiting to see Aunt Betty one more time?

After Aunt Betty arrived and after she had visited with Mom, she said, "My sister is not long for this world. She is all I have." My aunt could see the decline in her sister's health.

My grandparents had left this Earth many years ago, and my mother's only other sibling died very early in life. Aunt Betty and I were sitting on the front porch when my brother Tommy returned. His gait appeared altered as if he was dragging one leg.

"What is wrong with your leg, Tommy?" said Aunt Betty.

"Nothing. I just have this headache and I am tired. I have been working all day. I need to go home and take a nap," said Tommy.

"Well, go home and get some rest. Don't worry about Nita. We are here," said Aunt Betty.

"Do you want me to take you home, Tommy?" I asked.

"No, I can drive. It's just around the corner, and I am not that tired," said Tommy.

I climbed in the bed with Mom because I could not bear the thought of her not being here anymore. I talked to Mom at least four times a week, if not more, even before she had ever had a cancer diagnosis. My mom was my mother, but she was also my best friend. I would call her first to discuss things I was planning, like painting the interior of the house or planting flowers. Of course, I discussed it with my husband as well. But it was different having that conversation with Mom. She was taught to make a lot of her decorations herself—needlepoint, sewing draperies, and making quilts, just to mention a few of the things she did. The next morning, Mom was sitting up in bed, smiling.

"What has put that wonderful smile on your face?" I asked.

"I am the bride of Christ," said Mom. She smiled and nodded. I was unaware of that Christian reference, "bride of Christ." What I have since learned is that Christians referred to this as a mystic marriage in the New Testament. This "marriage" is seen as a union of the human soul with God. I could feel the peace Mom was experiencing, which was just another acknowledgment that my time with my mother was coming to an end. Sister Maria, a member of the Dominican Sisters of Peace in Kentucky, came by to visit with Mom, which was something that occurred frequently even before Mom was ill. They sat together talking and praying for an extended period of time.

Later that evening, the reverend came by to visit Mom, and he gave her communion. Someone from church would bring her communion weekly. I returned home feeling comforted by all the love being showered upon Mom. I wanted to stay at home with her, but I had a new boss who was unfamiliar with my work history. Each time I went home to visit my mother, my boss would call to see when I was returning to work. I decided I needed to return home.

After I was home for a week, Tommy called and said, "Mom was so weak, she was unable to get out of bed without help."

The hospice nurse and I touched base, and we agreed that Mom needed to be transferred to the hospital. Her care had reached the point of requiring two people and more assistive devices, which we were unable to provide at home. Once Mom arrived at the hospital, she was given IV fluids and antibiotics. As her condition improved, the doctor decided she need to continue physical therapy. That decision meant she would go to the nursing home. Ironically, the very place we had tried so hard to avoid is where she was now being admitted. Transportation was arranged to a facility thirty minutes from her home. She would be close to my nephews, who loved and respected their grandmother.

My nephews are grown adult men who still refer to Mom as "GrandNita." Mom was the pillar in all our eyes. I drove home to sign the necessary contracts and to be present. We decided to contact the funeral home to make arrangements as well, given the change in Mom's condition.

My mother had written instructions for her music selections and soloist. Once at the facility, Mom, Bobby, and I spoke with the administrator. Our plan was for her to stay there until she was stronger— just to be able to roll from side to side and stand with a walker. I was hopeful, but the nurse in me feared something different.

Over the next few weeks, Mom made some progress. She was going to physical therapy and receiving IV antibiotics for her urinary tract infection. My brother's seven sons would alternate visiting Mom almost daily, by their choice. They would call me and give me updates, but I knew they truly enjoyed that time they experienced with Mom. She told my nephews to make sure they looked out for my brother Bobby, because she knew he would take it hard. I remember Mrs. Goveart saying those exact words to me about her daughter.

Just as we thought Mom was making progress, her health made a sharp decline. Her respirations became more labored, and she was unable to get out of bed. The nursing home decided to transfer her to the hospital. Once I was notified, although crying and anxiously praying, I made my flight arrangements to Kentucky.

I tried to call my brother Tommy, but there was no answer. That was unusual; he always answered right away. I called my brother Bobby, who lived in the same town, just a few blocks over.

"Bobby, can you go check on Tommy? He did not answer his phone," I said.

"He is probably home sleeping. I don't want to go out right now. I just got home myself," said Bobby.

"I am sorry you are tired, but I am getting a bad feeling. I need you to go over there, please," I said.

"OK, I will call you when I get there," said Bobby.

The phone rang, and I heard Bobby's voice saying, "Bernice, there is an ambulance in Tommy's driveway. They are taking him to the hospital. He passed out. They found him face down on the kitchen floor. The door to his truck was open, and the kitchen door was propped open. Tommy's neighbor called her friend to go check on him because she didn't want to go to a man's house, being that she is an elderly woman. He found him and called the ambulance."

"Oh my God, Bobby I am so glad you went by his house. Otherwise, we wouldn't have known where he was," I said.

"They think he might have had a heart attack or hit his head on the paint can sitting next to the door. They are taking him to the hospital now," said Bobby.

By that morning, we knew Tommy had a brain tumor and had been flown to a trauma hospital sixty miles away. Oh my goodness—that is why he was having headaches and falling asleep so much. I thought it was because he was tired from working and trying to help take care of Mom. Both my mother and brother were admitted to the hospital on the same day.

Please, Lord, I know you think I have big shoulders, but please help my family.

Once my plane landed, I quickly gathered my luggage and headed off to the hospital. I stopped at the hospital in Louisville first to see Tommy. He could not be discharged or told of mother's declining health, as his own health was fragile at that point. He was in a neurology intensive care unit. I walked into his room, and I could see a bag of fluids hanging lower than his head, with serosanguineous drainage noted in the tubing.

Oh my goodness, I thought, *he has fluid draining from his brain*. I noticed there was 650cc of fluid in the bag.

"Hi, Tommy," I said.

He looked at me and said, "What are you doing here? Is Mom dead? Don't lie to me. I have got to get out of this hospital," said Tommy.

"Tommy, I needed to come see you and Mom. It was time for me to come home again." I stayed long enough to get him relaxed and calmed down, and then it was off to see Mom at the next hospital, thirty minutes away. En route to the hospital, I started crying. The gravity of it all had caught up with me. When I arrived in Mom's room, she opened her eyes briefly and acknowledged that I was present.

I embraced her; I was holding on so tightly, I realized I was making her feel uncomfortable. Mom did not talk much, nor did she eat. She only took sips of water. There was a knot in my stomach as I realized that the time had come for me to accept the fact that Mom was leaving me. I stood there, held her hands, and prayed. There was a knock on the door. The nurse entered with the social worker, whom I recognized because her mother had been my Girl Scout leader many years ago. Our families' farms were across from one another. Our mothers had stayed in contact with one another over the years. It was comforting to see her face. My brother Bobby and his son were sitting at Mom's bedside. I could see the hurt and pain in Bobby's eyes.

He said, "I have to go. I feel relieved now that you are here."

I planned to spend the night, so the nurse brought a Geri chair for me. The doctor had ordered an ultrasound of Mom's chest and lungs. The technician arrived and started performing the procedure at the bedside. I stepped out of the room to talk to the nurse to find out if Mom had received any pain medication, because she seemed distant. I knew what was happening, but I just wanted to make sure it was not the medication. I stayed at her bedside for the remainder of the night.

I held Mom's hands and prayed. I placed blessed oil on her, making the sign of the cross. When I looked at the area with oil on her chest, it was in the shape of a heart. I asked my nephew if he saw anything. He could see the shape of the heart as well. My nephew hugged me and then left after I settled in for the night and placed my chair next to her bed. I held her hand throughout the night.

Morning arrived, and I could hear that rattle in her throat. I asked the nurse for a Yankauer tip and suction kit. She paused and looked at me for a moment but then brought me the equipment. I explained to Mom what I was going to do.

Mom grabbed my hand and said, "What does it matter?"

I knew what that rattle meant, but I was having a hard time accepting it.

I just needed to stop being a nurse and be a daughter.

My sweet sister-in-law, Anna, arrived with my nephew to bring song and praise.

She started off by laughing and telling Mom, "Now, Mrs. Juanita, you cannot leave me here with these two. You know they are going to drive me crazy."

Then she proceeded to sing to Mom. Anna had a wonderful, soulful, soothing voice. She had a way of making everything make sense.

Anna said, "Go eat and take a break. I know you haven't left this room." She was right—I had not left the floor since I arrived.

I felt like I could use a break, but at the same time, I was torn about leaving. Eventually, I left the hospital. At the restaurant, I could not eat or enjoy my food. I just kept thinking, *What am I doing here?* I did not come 650 miles to sit in a restaurant. I came here to be with my mother in her time of need. I asked for the check and requested that my food be placed in carry-out boxes and headed back to the hospital.

I walked briskly to Mom's room. When I opened the door, I heard Anna's smooth voice lifting my mother's spirit up in song. But Mom was having agonal breathing. I scooped her up in my arms. I began to cry, and my nephew asked, "What's wrong?"

I could not speak the words. I thought, *I cannot say she is really leaving us.*

My nephew came to my side and said, "What's wrong? Is she gone?"

I could only nod at that moment. I was able to lay her down and adjust her as I would any of my patients. Mom had taken her last breath in my arms. My nephew and I embraced to console each other. I was so grateful that we were able to be at her side. I had no idea God would give me the gift of embracing my mother as she transitioned.

We contacted the nurse, and Anna began contacting our family. The nurse and doctor came to assess Mom. We all stood there, feeling the uncertainty of the moment. I felt as though my legs wanted to give away, but I knew we had to gather ourselves and leave. I felt a sense of gratitude for that final embrace and to have been present.

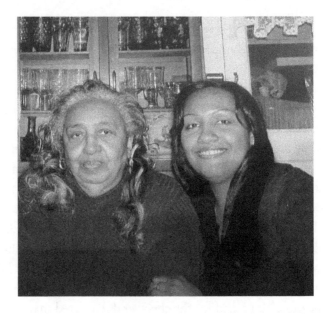

"And I saw a new heaven and a new earth: for the first heaven and the first earth were passed away; and there was no more sea.

And I John saw the holy city, New Jerusalem, coming down from God out of heaven, prepared as a bride adorned for her husband.

And I heard a great voice out of heaven saying, Behold, the tabernacle of God is with men, and he will dwell with them, and they shall be his people, and God himself shall be with them, and be their God.

And God shall wipe away all tears from their eyes, and there shall be no more death, neither sorrow, nor crying, neither shall there be any more pain for the former things are passed away.

And he that sat upon the throne said, Behold, I make all things new. And he said unto me, Write: for these words are true and faithful.

And he said unto me, it is done. I am Alpha and Omega, the beginning and the end. I will give unto him that is athirst of the fountain of the water freely." (Revelation 21:1–6, King James Version)

"To everything there is a season, and a time to every purpose under the heaven: A time to be born, and a time to die; A time to plant, and a time to pluck up that which is planted; A time to weep, and a time to laugh; A time to mourn, and a time to dance; A time to cast away stones, and a time to gather stones together; A time to embrace, and a time to refrain from embracing." (Ecclesiastes 3:1–2, 4–5, King James Version)

"Let us rejoice and be glad and give him glory! For the wedding of the Lamb has come, and his bride has made herself ready. Fine linen, bright and clean, was given to her to wear." (Revelation 19:7–8, New International Version)

"Is anyone among you sick? Let them call the elders of the church to pray over them and anoint them with oil in the name of the Lord. And the prayer of faith shall save the sick, and the Lord shall raise him up, and if he have committed sin, they shall be forgiven him." (James 5:14–15, King James Version)

My mom's favorite song was "His Eye Is on The Sparrow"

"Why should I feel discouraged
Why should the shadows come
Why should my heart be lonely
And long for heaven and home
When, when Jesus is my portion
My constant friend is he;
His eye is on the sparrow, And I know He watches me;
His eye is on the sparrow, and I know He watches me.
I sing because I'm happy, I said because I'm free,
For His eye is on the sparrow, and I know He watches me.
'Let not your heart be troubled,' His tender word I hear,
And resting on His goodness, I lose my doubts and fears;
Though by the path He leadeth, but one step I may see;
His eye is on the sparrow, and I know He watches me;
His eye is on the sparrow, and I know He watches me.
Whenever I am tempted, whenever clouds arise,
When songs give place to sighing, when hope within me dies,
I draw the closer to Him, from care He sets me free;
His eye is on the sparrow, and I know He watches me;
His eye is on the sparrow, and I know He watches me."

The premise of this song comes from the Bible verses Matthew 10:29–31, King James Version:

"Are not two sparrows sold for a farthing? And one of them shall not fall on the ground without your Father. But the very hairs of your head are all numbered. Fear ye not therefore, ye are more value than many sparrows."

After news of my mother's death was shared in the community, we began hearing knocks at my mother's back door. People said things like, "Hello. I just wanted you to know how much I appreciated your mother. I could come here and talk with her about anything, and I never heard it repeated."

There were so many people I didn't know who had a relationship with our mother. People even volunteered to be a part of her ceremony. All of this spoke volumes to the person she was and who I aspire to be. After my mother passed, I was never in the presence of someone dying. If a patient passed, it happened before or after my shift. I was grateful for that gift.

My mother believed in the use of homeopathic remedies since I was a child. She continued the use of echinacea even after her diagnosis, which I believe helped with the inflammation, one of the side effects of her disease.

My brother Tommy is currently living with a shunt in place. He was disappointed that he could not be present when Mom died or attend her funeral. He has since accepted her death and forgiven us for not telling him she was dying.

Our neighbors who own the family farm across from us are still my mother's neighbors. They are buried next to each other.

Somehow that just seems right.

CHAPTER 13

Upsilon Υυ: Clarification

Finding meaning in the mint of it all.

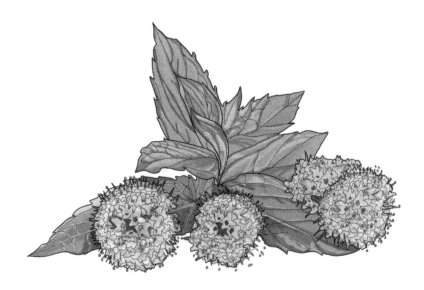

| Mint improves mental awareness and focus.[15]

The Greek letter *upsilon* means "pure, purified," and "purifying."

The clarification is to acknowledge the privilege it was to provide care for the patients who allowed me to be in their presence or worked a shift during their end of life. This allowed me to develop endurance, strength, and understanding of my own siblings' and family members' deaths.

While I was writing this book, some of my siblings and many other family members moved on to eternal life.

After my sister died, my daughter said to me one day, "Mom, you have to prepare yourself. You are the baby of the family, which means having the responsibility of helping them through their end-of-life care and preparing yourself for them to die."

So it seems the lesson was learned. My mother wanted me to show strength so that my children would learn how to deal with death. We acknowledge that each person's spirit and memories continue to live in our hearts—thereby they continue to live in us. Finding balance while grieving can be difficult, but having a support system is helpful. I am not saying I am a master at grieving or end-of-life care, but allowing your mind to focus on something that relieves your stress is important. Spirituality has always been a part of my life; it gives me peace after reading the Bible or reciting a prayer.

Ubuntu is a philosophy of African tribes that can be summed up as, "I am because you are." How can one of us be happy if all the others are sad? This concept embraces the philosophy that we are all dependent on community, connection, and caring. In essence, if we could imagine ourselves in the position of someone else and experience what they are going through, our world would be different.

As health-care providers, imagine that person lying in that bed as your mother, sister, aunt, brother, father, or uncle. With that being said, we celebrate new life, but the end of life has just as much importance because it is a person's final acts, words, or desires before leaving this Earth. Our presence as family, friends, acquaintances, or health-care providers is important. We are not just individuals; we are dependent upon each other.

It does not matter what race, belief, or disbelief of spirituality. Being present during someone's end of life is difficult, but if you have the fortitude to show up, you may learn you possess a strength you were unaware of. There is always someone willing to help you and your significant other through the process. Sometimes, we are not given the opportunity because of a sudden loss, but the power of prayer may give you or others comfort for the loss of your loved one.

You can also write that person a letter or journal about your feelings to cope with the loss. All the things you are experiencing require you to focus on what is happening in that moment. Our perceptions of death may and may not be true. Being present allows you to define those perceptions with reality.

If you are a health-care provider, allow yourself to be present in the moment and examine your patients and their families, if they are present. You can determine when and where you need to interject. For example, if the family is having a disagreement in the presence of the patient and you see signs of distress in your patient, it is acceptable to ask the family to leave the room. Explain why you are asking them to leave, and if you feel so inclined, help them understand the power of their words in a patient's presence.

There is no need to be rude, because it is not beneficial to the patient or to them. Help them see that discord is causing their loved one stress. The family can then hopefully come to some resolution, or you can provide them a space away from where the patient is resting to continue their conversation. Helping the family come to terms with their loved one's imminent death is vital to providing a pleasant environment for that patient, the family, and the other patients on the unit due to noise level.

Sometimes, family members are so distraught that they show their passion in unbecoming ways. If they had it to do all over again, they probably would have desired not to act that way. I have seen a patient's body language change from peaceful to anxious, even when the patient is unresponsive.

But as the nurse, it is your duty to focus on the comfort of your patient. Most of the time, people understand the reasoning behind the request, but if you anticipate disruptive behavior, you can always call security to have them on the unit just in case. It is important to understand that the final gift you can give to someone is to help them be in a peaceful and comfortable state before his or her departure from this Earth.

When I began caring for end-of-life patients, I was exhausted by the time they died because I understand the pain of loving and losing someone dear to your heart.

However, as time went on, I learned to manage my time and stress, and my plan of care improved.

Enjoy people, and don't be afraid of taking care of someone who has life choices to make. Experiencing what that patient is going through provides you with the opportunity to grow as a person. It provides you with potential insight for your own life choices. So resolve those conflicts, or have that discussion with whomever you may need to. Achieving peace within yourself is priceless. Peace comes from within; it is not something that someone can give you. You cannot change what has happened in the past. The past is the past, so do not try to fix it or change it; it is done. Move forward and try to live your best life.

I am very grateful for the experiences, knowledge, and exposure I have had in being a part of the team of managing a patient's care, cultural practices, and end-of-life journey. I am not perfect—none of us are—but we can all strive to be the best version of ourselves.

> "These things I have spoken unto you, that in me ye might have peace. In the world ye shall have tribulation: but be of good cheer; I have overcome the world." (John 16:33, King James Version)

> "Owe no man anything, but to love one another: for he that loveth one another has fulfilled the law." (Romans 13:8, King James Version)

1) Determine your patient's acceptance of their disease process and impending end of life.

2) Determine their spiritual beliefs and contact the appropriate religious affiliation if the patient desires.
3) Ask if there is something that needs to be completed.
4) Determine if there is someone they would like to have present.
5) Address pain management, oxygen needs, and anxiety level.
6) Contact the palliative care team if patient desires.
7) Promote comfort by offering nutrition as tolerated, change linens, oral care, and maintain hygienic needs.
8) Contact required agencies per your facilities protocol (e.g., organ donation).

A PRAYER OF SAINT FRANCIS OF ASSISI

Lord make me an instrument of your peace.
Where there is hatred, let me sow love.
Where there is injury, pardon,
Where there is doubt, faith,
Where there is despair, hope,
Where there is darkness, light,
and where there is sadness, joy.
O Divine Master,
grant that I may not so much seek to be consoled,
as to console;
To be understood, as to understand,
To be loved, as to love;
For it is in giving that we receive
It is in pardoning that we are pardoned.
And it is in dying that we are born to eternal life.

The hands of a nurse embrace the newly born infant,
stroke the forehead.
The hands of a nurse wipe the tears, sweat,
and many other excrements away.

The hands of a nurse insert the tubes to
remove the fluids and then remove
those same tubes when it is time.
The hands of a nurse apply nasal cannula or oxygen mask to supply the
oxygen required to breathe.
The hands of a nurse hold their patients
hands as they transition from this
life to the next.

RESOURCES

According to the Kübler-Ross model, which was established in 1969, referenced from the book, On Death and Dying, there are **five stages of grief**:

1) **Denial**: Shock, fear, confusion, avoidance, and elation. "I feel fine." "This can't be happening, not to me."
2) **Anger**: Frustration, anxiety, irritation. "Why Me?" "It's not fair!" "How can this happen to me?"
3) **Bargaining**: Telling one's own story, struggling to find meaning, and reaching out to others. Guilt is also common during this stage. "Just let me live to see my children graduate."
4) **Depression**: Overwhelmed, helplessness, hostility, and fight. "I'm so sad; why bother with anything?" "I'm going to die, so what's the point?"
5) **Acceptance**: Exploring options, putting a new plan in place. Moving on doesn't mean the grief is over; it just means we are accepting of it at this particular time. "It's going to be okay." "I can't fight it; I may as well prepare for it."

The National Alliance for Grieving Children (NAGC)

The NAGC in Lubbock, Texas, provides a list of support services providers for each state. There are also in-school bereavement programs. (866) 432-1542
https://childrengrieve.org

Hospice Foundation of America

Hospice provides medical care and support to a person who has been determined to have six months or less to live, as determined by a physician. The plan is to provide comfortable living, not to cure illness.

Hospice care also provides short-term relief to family caregivers to avoid "caregiver burnout." They can also provide necessary information about tough decisions for end-of-life care such as mechanical breathing, use of IVs for hydration and feeding tubes for nutrition, or choosing to discontinue treatment to allow comfort. Grief counseling for patients and loved ones is also available.
https://hospicefoundation.org

Five Wishes

Five Wishes is a document that allows you to make personal, emotional, and spiritual decisions while you are still mentally able to. This document will communicate your desires to your health-care providers. Five Wishes was started by Jim Towey, after he had served as legal counsel for Mother Teresa. He was a full-time live-in volunteer at her home for AIDS patients in Washington, DC.

Wish 1

The person I want to make health-care decisions for me when I can't make them for myself.

Wish 2

My wish for the kind of medical treatment I want or don't want.

Wish 3

My wish for how comfortable I want to be.

Wish 4

My wish for how I want people to treat me.

Wish 5

My wish for what I want my loved ones to know.

After you complete five wishes, keep it nearby so you or someone else can find it when you need it. Give a copy to your doctor so it can be placed in your medical record; if you are admitted to a hospital, take a copy for their records.

(888)5-WISHES or (888)594-7437
www.FiveWishes.org

Alexandra Hartwell's Drawing   Contact information: <u>alexb0731@gmail.com</u>

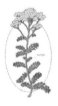 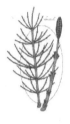 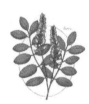 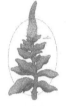 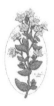

Keri Kubota's Drawings   Contact information:<<u>keri@ourgardencollective.com</u>>

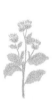  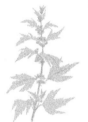 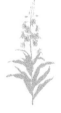

Tiara Butler Drawings   Contact information:
DesignsByTiaraB@gmail

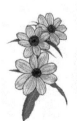

APPENDIX

achurchnearyou.com. The Chaplet of Divine Mercy.
Anointing of The Sick. Holy Bible, The New American Bible. Kansas, Fireside Bible Publishers. 2002 Encyclopedic Dictionary, page 12.

CA: a cancer journal for clinicians. 2018 May;68(3):182–196. Published online 2018 Mar 30.NIHMSID: NIHMS948664
https://www.ncbi.nlm.nih.gov>pmc
Optimal Pain Management for Patients with Cancer in the Modern Era

English definitions are derived from Webster's New Universal Unabridged Dictionary (New York: Barnes & Noble,1996).

Gutgsell, Michael, J.C.D, Peter, S.T.D., J.C.D., Third Order, Valentine J. Encyclopedic Dictionary, Holy Bible, The New American Bible. Copyright 1981, By Devore & Sons, INC. Kansas 116.

Herbal Active Ingredients: An Emerging Potential for the Prevention and treatment of Papillary Thyroid Carcinoma. Yang Y, Chen Q, Yu WY, Zhang HH, Zhong YS, Zhang SZ, Wang JF, YU CH. https://doi.org/10.1155/2020/1340153 (Chapter 9)

Hunhu/Ubuntu, Internet Encyclopedia of Philosophy.
https:// iep.utm.edu>hunhu

Lidell, Henry George, Scott, Robert. Definitions of Greek words. Greek-English Lexicon. Ninth Edition (Oxford: Oxford University Press, 1996, first published 1843).

http://www.thellf.org. The Living Legacy Foundation. A non-profit organization dedicated to saving and enhancing lives through organ and tissue donation.

Proppe, Catherine A. Greek Alphabet: Unlock the Secrets (Michigan: Edwards Brothers - Malloy Copyright 2 0 1 7) 5,13,31,22,41,45,64,85 ,89,108,133,115.

The National Center for Complementary and Integrative Health clearinghouse. The NCCIH clearinghouse provides information on NCCIH and complementary and integrative health approaches, including publications and searches of Federal databases of scientific and medical literature. Toll-free in the United States: 1-888-644-6226 tty (for deaf and hard-of-hearing callers): 1-866-464-3615 Website: https:// nccih.nih.gov/Email: info@nccih.nih.gov

Li CY, Lee SC, Lai WL, Chang KF, Huang XF, Hung PY, Lee CP, Hsieh MC, Tsai NM. Cell Cycle Arrest and Apoptosis induction by Juniperius communis extract in Esophageal squamous cell carcinoma through activation of p53-induced apoptosis pathway. Food Science & Nutrition. 2020 December 30;9(2):1088-1098. doi:10.1002/fsn3.2084. PMID: 33598192; PMCID:PMC7866587 (Chapter 2).

YS, Zhang SZ, Wang Jf, Yu CH. Herbal Active Ingredients: An Emerging Potential for the Prevention and Treatment of Papillary Thyroid Carcinoma. Biomed Res Int. 2020 Jan 31;2020:1340153. doi:10.1155/2020/1340153. PMID:32090065; PMCID: PMC7013308.

Kubler-Ross, MD, Elizabeth. On Death and Dying. TOUCHSTONE. New York, NY. Copyright 1969.

Mohanty I, Arya D. S, Gupta S. K.. Effect of Curcuma longa and Ocimum sanctum on myocardial apoptosis in experimentally induced myocardial ischemic-reperfusion injury. BMC Complement Altern Med. 2006;6:3 (Chapter 1).

Schepetkin IA, Ramstead AG, Kirkpotina LN, Voyich JM, Jutila MA, Quinn MT. Therapuetic Potential of Polyphenols from Epilobium Angustifolium (Fireweed). Phytother Res. 2016 Aug; 30(8):

1287-1297. Published online 2016 May 24. doi:10.1002/ptr.5648. PMCID:PMC5045895

NIHMSID: NIHMS818633 PMID:27215200 (Chapter 3)

Chiavari-Frederico MO, Barbosa LN, Carvalho Dos Santos I, et al. Antimicrobial activity of Asteraceae Species against bacterial pathogens isolated from postmenopausal women. PLoS One. 2020;15(1):e0227023.31905207 (Chapter4)

Mohsen Hamidpour, Rafie Hamidpour, Sohelia Hamidpour, and Mina Shahlari. J Tradit Complement Med. 2014 Apr-Jun; 4(2):82-88. doi:10.4103/2225-4110.130373. PMCID: PMC4003706 PMID: 24860730 (Chapter 5)

José Blanco-Salas, Maria P. Hortigon-Vinagre, Diana Morales-Jadan, and Trinidad Ruiz-Tellez. Biology (Basel). 2021 Jul; 10(7): 618 Published online 2021 Jul 2. Doi:10.3390/biology10070618 PMCID: PMC8301161 PMID: 34356473 (Chapter 6)

LiverTox: Clinical and Research Information on Drug Induced Liver Injury [Internet]. Bethesda (MD): National Institute of Diabetes and Digestive and Kidney Diseases; 2012- Horsetail. [updated 2022 Jul 25]. PMID: 35998247 (Chapter 7)

Denisa Batir-Marin, Monica Boev, Oana Cioanca, Cornelia Mircea, Ana Flavia Burlec, Galba jean Beppe, Adrian Spac, Andreia Corciova, Lucian Hritcu, and Monica hancianu. U.S. National Institute of Health Molecules. 2021 May; 26(9):2565. Published online 2021 apr 28. Doi: 10.3390/molecules26092565 PMCID: PMC8124630 PMID: 33924900 (Chapter 7)

Oleh Koshovyi, Ain Raal, Igor Kireyev, Nadiya Tryshchuk, Tetiana Ilina, Yevhen Romanenko, Sergiy M Kovalenko, and Natalya Bunyatyan. Plants (Basel). 2021 Feb; 10(2):230. Published online 2021 Jan 25. Doi:

10.3390/plants10020230 PMCID: PMC7911030 PMID: 33503956 (Chapter 8)

Pro Natl Acad Sci USA. 2017 Jan 31; 114(5):974-979. Published online 2017 Jan 17. Doi: 10.1073/pnas.1612901114 PMCID: PMC5293046 PMID: 28096378 Biochemistry. Sibongile Mafu, Prema Sambandaswami Karunanithi, Teresa Ann Palazzo, Brownyn Lee Harrod, Selina Marakana Rodriguez, Iris Natalie Mollhoff, Terrence Edward O'Brien, Shen Tong, Oliver Fiehn, Dean Tantillo, Jorg Bohlmann, and Philipp Zerbe (Chapter 9).

Phytother Res. 2018 Dec; 32(12): 2323-2339. Published online 2018 Aug 17. Doi: 10.1002/ptr.6178 PMCID: PMC7167772 PMID: 30117204 Guilia Pastorino, Laura Cornara, Sonia Soares, Francisca Rodrigues, and M. Beatriz P.P. Oliveria (Chapter 10).

Klemow KM, Bartlow A., Crawford J, et al. Medical Attributes of St. John's Wort (Hypericum perforatum) In:Benzie IFF, Wachtel-Galor S, editors. Herbal Medicine:Biomolecular and Clinical Aspects. 2nd edition. Boca Raton (FL): CRC Press/Taylor & Francis; 2011. Chapter 11.

Pharmacogn Rev. 2015 Jan-Jun; 9(17): 63-72. Doi: 10.4103/0973-7847.156353 PMCID: PMC4441164 PMID: 26009695 Azadeh Manayi, Mahdi Vazirian, and Soodabeh Saeidnia (Chapter 12).

Moss M, Hewitt S, Moss L, Wesnes K. Modulation of cognitive performance and mood by aromas of peppermint and ylang-ylang. Int J Neurosci. 2008 Jan;118(1):59-77. Doi: 10.1080/00207450601042094. PMID: 18041606 (Chapter 13).

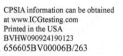
CPSIA information can be obtained
at www.ICGtesting.com
Printed in the USA
BVHW090924190123
656605BV00006B/263